THE CLOSED TREATMENT
OF COMMON FRACTURES

THE
CLOSED TREATMENT
OF
COMMON FRACTURES

BY

JOHN CHARNLEY
B.Sc., M.B., F.R.C.S.

Orthopædic Surgeon, Manchester Royal Infirmary; Orthopædic Surgeon,
The Park Hospital, Davyhulme; Orthopædic Surgeon, Wrightington
Hospital; Honorary Lecturer in Orthopædics, Manchester University;
Late Hunterian Professor, Royal College of Surgeons.

FOURTH EDITION

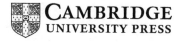

CAMBRIDGE
UNIVERSITY PRESS

CAMBRIDGE UNIVERSITY PRESS
Cambridge, New York, Melbourne, Madrid, Cape Town, Singapore, São Paulo, Delhi

Cambridge University Press
The Edinburgh Building, Cambridge CB2 8RU, UK

www.cambridge.org
Information on this title: www.cambridge.org/9780521682879

First Published 1950
This edition published 1999
Reprinted 2005
Reprinted by Cambridge University Press 2005
Third printing 2008

Printed in the United Kingdom at the University Press, Cambridge

A catalogue record for this publication is available from the British Library

ISBN 978-0-521-68287-9 paperback

TO
MY TEACHER
SIR HARRY PLATT

ACKNOWLEDGMENTS

IT gives me great pleasure to thank Mr H. Osmond-Clarke, C.B.E., F.R.C.S., for reading my original manuscript and for the numerous kindly and constructive suggestions which he has made.

My thanks are due also to Dr R. G. W. Ollerenshaw and Mr J. Kilshaw of the staff of the Department of Medical Illustration at the Manchester Royal Infirmary, without whose skill this book could hardly have been undertaken.

The Publishers of the *Lancet*, the American and British Editors of the *Journal of Bone and Joint Surgery*, and Messrs Butterworth have kindly allowed me to reproduce illustrations from articles of mine previously published by them.

CONTENTS

FOREWORD
TO THE GOLDEN JUBILEE EDITION

BY

CHRISTOPHER FAUX

Former pupil, consultant orthopædic surgeon and
Chairman of the Trustees of The John Charnley Trust.

THIS monograph was written fifty years ago by John Charnley when he was in his late thirties. Always a highly-practical orthopædic surgeon with great clarity of thought, he combined his vast experience of fracture treatment gleaned from industrial Manchester and service in World War II to produce this work which is full of basic commonsense. It should be compulsory reading for all those involved in learning the art of fracture management and all students of orthopædic surgery.

Open reduction of fractures and internal fixation is commonplace and successful in many cases in the 1990's, but is not the total answer to fracture treatment. In many parts of the world, initial treatent, and frequently the final treatment, is by closed methods, and this book has become the bible for many isolated and lonely junior orthopædic surgeons in remote areas.

The basic principles described are a benchmark and, like the Charnley hip, a gold standard from which to start if progress is to be made in the future.

The John Charnley Trust has decided to reprint this Golden Jubilee edition of *The Closed Treatment of Common Fractures* for the next generation of orthopædic surgeons in training, to coincide with the Millennium.

The aims, objectives and achievements of The John Charnley Trust are contained in the final page of this edition.

January, 1999

CHRISTOPHER FAUX

FOREWORD

BY

SIR HARRY PLATT

Professor of Orthopædic Surgery, University of Manchester

THE treatment of fractures and dislocations is one of the oldest forms of surgical handicraft, and the influence of many of the principles and procedures expounded in such clear detail in the corpus of Hippocratic texts can be witnessed in the practice of casualty surgery at the present day. Thus Hippocrates taught the importance of the early reduction of deformity, and the value of continued traction as a means of maintaining correct alignment of the limb. But despite the antiquity of the theoretical knowledge thus available, every young surgeon in his turn, when first confronted with responsibility for the ' setting ' of fractures, has to acquire his own sense of manipulative skill, usually by the process of trial and error. In this stimulating monograph Mr Charnley has sought to illuminate some of the obscurities of the mechanics of fracture treatment, and he has succeeded, in a most vivid fashion, in creating by means of text and illustration a series of mental pictures—a frame of reference, so to say—whereby the young surgeon can get the ' feel ' of a fracture ; first the anatomy of the displacement, and then that confident ' clinical sense ' of precise correction of the deformity which follows a skilful manipulative act of reduction. Mr Charnley has also incorporated in this book his original observations on the genesis and prevention of joint stiffness ; his well-known ingenious work on the design and uses of the walking caliper ; and not least in importance, an invaluable chapter in which he presents a critical study of the various types of modern plaster-of-Paris technique.

Although the author has addressed his message primarily to the young casualty surgeon there is much in this monograph which will persuade the experienced orthopædic surgeon to re-examine some of his most cherished presuppositions.

HARRY PLATT.

PREFACE TO THE FIRST EDITION

THIS book is written primarily for the resident casualty surgeon. In Britain this resident appointment is usually held by young men whose practical experience, for obvious reasons, cannot match their theoretical knowledge. It is possible for such casualty officers to be fully conversant with modern textbooks of fracture treatment and yet be unable with any degree of certainty to reduce many of the simple fractures. I believe that this follows from the fact that in many large textbooks the space devoted to the detailed description of technique in the treatment of the common fractures is disproportionately small. An important step, on which might depend the whole success of a reduction, can be overlooked if it is concealed within one sentence. The full significance of many sentences in standard textbooks is often only realised on reading them again at a later date, when one has learned to reduce fractures by practical experience.

I have therefore in this small volume endeavoured to describe in detail what I consider to be the essential steps in the closed reduction of the common fractures, and at a length proportionate to the importance of the matter. No attempt has been made to write a comprehensive textbook but, by emphasising various mechanical features common to the reduction of certain fractures (which might almost be regarded as principles) it is hoped that the student may learn to apply these to the successful reduction of rare fractures whenever he encounters them.

The ease with which perfect reductions can be obtained by closed methods *when the injury is fresh* makes it especially important that the casualty officer should be skilful enough to take full advantage of being on the spot when the patient is first admitted to hospital.

It is possible that some persons are more naturally equipped for acquiring manipulative skill than others, but it is unlikely that there is any special gift which cannot be conscientiously acquired by everyone. The essential difficulty in performing a closed reduction can usually be traced to the surgeon not having a clear mental picture of what he is attempting to do. In these circumstances a series of manipulative movements is carried out as a ritual and an X-ray is then taken ' to see if it is reduced.' If, then, the fracture is not reduced the operator is nonplussed ; *he does not know what to do, having learned nothing from his previous attempt*. In the following chapters I have tried to create pictures for the surgeon to visualise in his mind's eye ; it must be confessed that some of these mental pictures may be more symbolic than true representations of the facts, but this approach has helped me to improve my own results, and those who attempt to follow can make their own images starting from this groundwork.

It should be the aim of a good manipulative surgeon *to know that a fracture has been reduced by his sense of touch without utter dependence on X-ray* ; it is possible to acquire this faculty for the Pott's, Colles', supracondylar fracture of the humerus, and the Bennett's fracture with some degree of certainty.

Contrary to popular ideas, the operative treatment of fractures is much simpler than is the non-operative. At operation the fracture lies open for all to see, and the mechanical procedures which may be needed are obvious in the extreme; yet modern textbooks often devote many chapters to minute descriptions of these self-evident facts.

In addition to its aim of guiding the young fracture surgeon, another motive for writing this book arose out of a recent visit to the United States of America. It became apparent to a British visitor that interest in the operative treatment of fractures was there tending to supersede interest in non-operative treatment, except, of course, where open methods were manifestly impossible. One obvious reason for this different viewpoint was economic; any method was likely to be favoured which enables the duration of hospital in-patient stay to be shortened. But it seemed that another reason for the trend towards open reduction in the United States of America and Canada might be that good operative techniques were being unfairly contrasted with poor manipulative techniques. But the appearance of scientific precision which is always associated with operative methods is often only superficial; this apparent precision will not alter the convictions of the manipulative surgeon and will not blind him to the ill-effects of many operative interventions on the blood supply of bone fragments and the process of normal callus formation. For this reason **an attempt is here made to re-emphasise the non-operative method, and to show that far from being a crude and uncertain art, the manipulative treatment of fractures can be resolved into something of a science.**

In order to carry out the conservative method adequately it is first necessary to revive interest in the perfection of plaster-of-Paris technique. For this the surgeon must discipline himself to a period of apprenticeship.

In the chapter devoted to the fractured femur I have set down an exposition of the Thomas method as I have used it in the last seven years. For many people this chapter may be of no more than historical interest as showing the degree to which a method used by H. O. Thomas in 1860 can be developed by the year 1949; but to my mind the method is one of extreme importance because, even if not practised, it illustrates certain principles in the mechanics of fracture treatment which are valid, though not so obviously, in other parts of the body and for this reason it is important that the method should be included in any training curriculum.

JOHN CHARNLEY.

Manchester, 1950.

PREFACE TO THE THIRD EDITION

IN this third edition I have persisted in my attempt to write a book on the conservative treatment of fractures which at one and the same time would be a vade-mecum for the junior man and an interesting treatise for the experienced surgeon. It might be considered that these two objectives are incompatible, and that it would have been better to have written a simple textbook for the junior and to have reserved my ponderings on the nature of fracture repair for a separate monograph. In the training of young surgeons I believe that the attempt to foster the habit of making clinical observations and questioning accepted beliefs ought to start from the earliest moment. There is still a great deal of fundamental information concerning the healing of fractures waiting to be deduced, by the process of logic and close reasoning, from clinical facts collected in the operating theatre and out-patient department.

There is a tendency to imagine that serious research nowadays can only come out of a laboratory, and that contributions from the pure act of thinking on clinical facts ended with the great clinicians of the past. The old clinicians had their faculties for observation by sight and touch heightened by the absence of X-rays and laboratory tests. But though the clinical acumen of the old observers was greater than ours, it was frequently offset by a strain of credulity, which is apparent in a different form among clinicians to-day. In the past the clinical philosopher was credulous because he was the victim of inherited beliefs, but to-day our credulity lies in the accuracy which we attribute to our special research tools, such as the electron microscope. We must not forget that sight and touch together make the greatest clinical faculty of all, namely, commonsense. As an instance of this I venture to suggest that the recent failure of ' bone glue ' could have been predicted from the facts of blood-supply in the process of fracture repair and that this conclusion could have been reached by arguments from the depth of an armchair without ever resorting to trials on the human subject.

As in the second edition, the chapter on fractures of the shaft of the tibia, of any in this book, has given me the greatest difficulty in writing. There are many fractures of the tibia for which conservative treatment is not adequate by itself and redisplacement of the fragments takes place after what initially was a satisfactory reduction. For these I am now recommending that, in selected cases, conservative treatment should be reinforced by a Rush-type nail and I have attempted to explain my reasons for choosing this particular type of imperfect fixation.

JOHN CHARNLEY.

Manchester, 1961.

CHAPTER ONE

CONSERVATIVE VERSUS OPERATIVE METHODS

IT is over thirty years since Arbuthnot Lane published his *Operative Treatment of Fractures*; but we still cannot compare conservative and operative principles from the viewpoint of basic science because the fundamental nature of fracture repair still eludes us. The best we can do is to compare the results of clinical practice; but there are so many variables (comminution, sepsis, mechanical details of the operation, blood supply, level of fracture, different observers, etc.) that a series of one or two hundred cases, which is a large series for any one operator, is soon reduced to statistical insignificance. Attempts to control the conditions of the fracture by using experimental animals have yielded nothing of importance compared with what we have learned ' the hard way' by developing operative techniques on the human subject.

The followers of Lane and Sherman believed that the failures of internal fixation would ultimately be eliminated by improved technique. We now know that internal splints are exposed to truly enormous forces and are subject to the phenomenon of failure by fatigue. Improvements in the design of plates and screws have reduced, but not eliminated, the mechanical failures which were common when techniques derived from the woodworker were used. The change to using electrolytically inert metals has only slightly diminished our problems, though there is no excuse for returning to the brass screws and reactive steel plates with which Lane himself achieved sufficient success to establish the method.

But despite improved technology, delayed union after internal fixation is still encountered. Immediately after any form of internal fixation there starts a race against time, between the bridging of the fracture gap by osseous union and the tendency for the mechanical fixation to loosen its attachment to the bone as a consequence of the millions of reversals of stress and strain which occur during the two or three months of convalescence. If osseous union has bridged the fracture line before the fixation becomes loose, then all will be well, but if union is delayed either the metal will fatigue and break (Fig. 1) or bending of the fixation will ensue (Fig. 2). It is unprofitable to argue that these failures are merely the results of inadequate fixation or that they could have been prevented by better engineering. In the two cases illustrated the surgeons were satisfied with the rigidity of the fixation at the time of operation. Blame should not therefore be transferred to defective fixation; the fault lies in the failure of osteogenesis to bridge the gap in the time during which mechanical fixation can reasonably be expected to hold firm. It will be one of the themes of this monograph that by open operation, the denuding of bone ends of periosteum in the case of cortical bone, or the prevention of collapse of fragments towards each other in the case of cancellous bone, carries

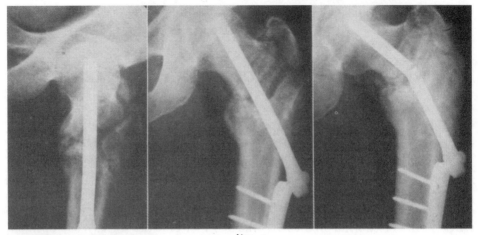
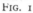

FIG. 1

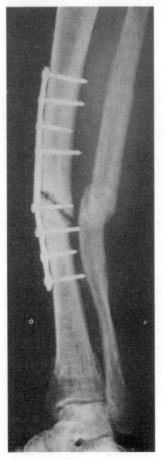

Fig. 1.—Fatigue fracture of nail ten months after operation. Despite transmission of body weight the fracture remained distracted. This fracture in cancellous bone demands compression, not distraction. Spontaneous filling of a gap in cancellous bone is a slow process.

Fig. 2.—Failure to bridge the fracture line. Rigid fixation was obtained at the original operation. There was initially no significant gap between the bone ends.

FIG. 2

with it the serious risk of artificially depressing osteogenic activity, and that this therefore invites the loosening or breakage of fixation before union can take over. An attempt will be made to emphasise the biological background to fracture repair and the dominating role of blood supply in the healing of bones.

THE NATURE OF FRACTURE REPAIR

The development of conservative or operative methods must be based on our knowledge of fracture repair. I believe that there are fundamental differences between the process of union in cancellous bone and cortical bone, and I will therefore describe these separately. Because of certain difficulties in terminology, before one can describe processes of fracture repair it is necessary to define precisely the use of certain histological terms.

DEFINITIONS

It is important to understand what is meant by the terms *woven bone* and *lamellar bone* (which is the terminology recommended by S. L. Baker) because though the two tissues themselves are absolutely distinct and easily recognisable, the variations in terminology in current literature are very confusing.

Woven bone is the bone of 'provisional' or 'temporary' callus. It is rapidly produced—often being in evidence histologically three or four days after fracture. Histologically the osteocytes are distributed through it in a rather irregular fashion like currants in a bun. It is called woven bone because the collagen fibres which

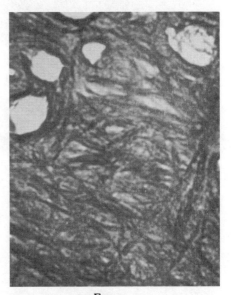

FIG. 3

Showing irregular arrangement of fibres in woven bone which constitutes callus. (×550.) (*Professor S. L. Baker's specimen.*

run through the osseous matrix are arranged in an irregular network though, strictly speaking, the appearance is more that of a 'felt' than a woven textile (Fig. 3). Woven bone is essentially a temporary tissue, being later removed and replaced. It is the medium of 'clinical union.' Woven bone develops in spindle-celled fibrous tissue as a precursor. The bony matrix is first seen appearing as an amorphous intercellular substance, between the fibres connecting the spindle cells (Fig. 4), staining with eosin more densely than the adjacent intercellular material. As the matrix increases in amount the spindle cells swell up and become incorporated to form the 'osteocytes.' This process is thus eminently suitable for the bridging of gaps between bone ends, because the spindle-celled tissue, by reason of its flexibility, has no difficulty in maintaining continuity in the presence of a certain amount of movement. It is not difficult to see how the matrix

3

can harden by taking up calcium and so immobilise the tissues to which it is connected.

Lamellar bone, on the other hand, is the permanent bone of the mature trabeculæ and the shafts of long bones. Lamellar bone is laid down in orderly layers (Fig. 5) and the osteocytes tend to be distributed regularly between the layers (more like a sandwich than a bun !). The fibre structure of each layer is

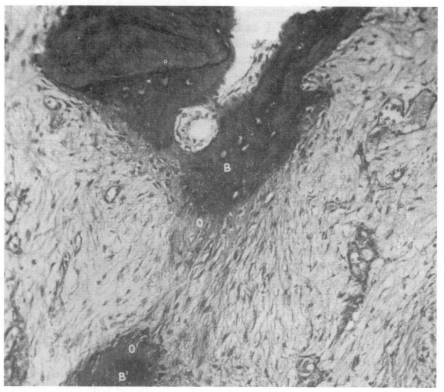

FIG. 4

The start of a fibrous trabecula composed of strands of collagenous substance with amorphous intercellular substance appearing between them. The fibres are streaming from one fragment of adult cancellous bone to another, and in so doing are crossing the line of arthrodesis. The inter-cellular substance is seen as a dark zone passing vertically down the centre of this illustration.

not an irregular felt-work as it is in woven bone but has a parallel arrangement, and in each layer the direction of the fibres crosses the direction of adjacent layers at an angle to give a ' ply ' structure of very great strength. It is obvious that this complicated structure needs time for its deposition—unlike the hurried production of woven bone. In this connection another fundamental difference distinguishes the process of deposition of lamellar bone from woven bone—*i.e.*, it is essential for there to be a solid framework on which the first layer of lamellar bone can be deposited before it can proceed to build up its multiple layers. Lamellar bone cannot be deposited in fibrous tissue and cannot therefore bridge

4

a moving gap spanned only by fibrous tissue. The solid framework on which lamellar bone is normally deposited is the woven bone of callus which has formed a temporary scaffold, and which is removed when the lamellar bone has acquired an adequate thickness. Later still, and continuing slowly over a long period of time, the first layers of lamellar bone are removed by osteoclasts and more lamellar bone is deposited on adjacent lamellæ in order to adjust the architecture of the trabeculæ to the forces acting on them in accordance with Wolff's Law.

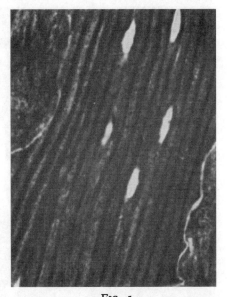

FIG. 5

Showing orderly arrangement in layers of lamellar bone. This constitutes mature bone no matter whether cortical or cancellous. (×980.) (*Professor S. L. Baker's specimen.*)

The Union of Cancellous Bone

Arthrodesis of the knee joint has presented a valuable source of human histological material for studying the healing of cancellous bone, described in detail elsewhere (Charnley and Baker, 1952; Charnley, 1953).

The observation which I think is the most significant in relation to the healing of fractures in cancellous bone was made on a biopsy four weeks after arthrodesis of a knee. In this particular case the surfaces of cancellous bone, produced by resection of the joint with a saw, were experimentally reduced to a small area of contact by making one of the bone ends wedge-shaped (Fig. 6). The knee had united solidly (under compression) four weeks after the operation, and the histology and microradiography of the biopsy are illustrated in Figs. 7, A and B, and 8, A, B and C. It is at once obvious that there has been very satisfactory union at the point of intimate contact; but the feature which is most significant in its bearing on fracture treatment is that *there is no evidence of ' callus' on the cut surfaces which are widely separated.* This is particularly well seen in the microradiograph. Histological examination of the cut ends of the trabeculæ on opposite sides of the gap shows only the faintest trace of the cellular activity which precedes the appearance of woven bone in these human biopsy specimens.

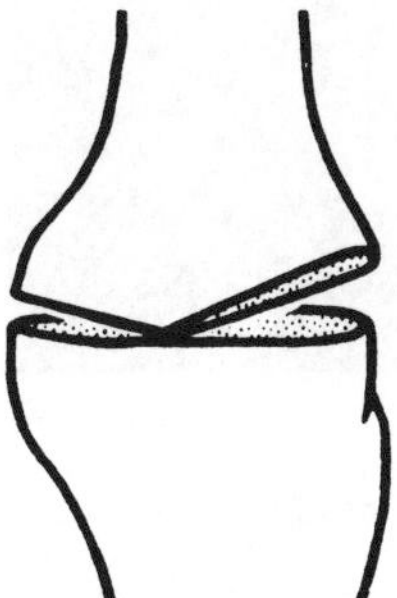

FIG. 6

Showing shape of surfaces in contact in knee arthrodesis described in text.

This observation, confirmed by the behaviour of other biopsy specimens, came to me as a very considerable surprise. I had been brought up to believe that cancellous bone was a highly osteogenic substance and that empty spaces between cancellous surfaces (as, for instance, in a foot stabilisation operation) would rapidly fill with new bone. I now believe that cancellous bone, even with an intact blood supply, has in fact a very restricted form of osteogenic activity. Cancellous bone

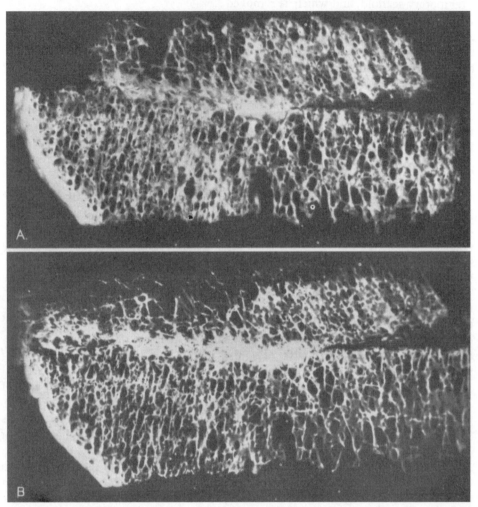

FIG. 7

Longitudinal section of coring from the 'crucial' experiment. A (*top*), Undecalcified, digested, specimen photographed by visible light (1 mm. thick slice). B (*bottom*), Microradiograph of same slice prior to digestion with trypsin. Note density of new bone maximal at site of maximal pressure and tailing off posteriorly where the pressure is less. Note absence of callus in gap where pressure is absent. Note absence of new bone on cut surfaces of the gap where there is no pressure and therefore no incentive to osteogenesis. Specimen at four weeks. Magnification approximately × 4.

certainly can unite very rapidly, but it unites rapidly only at the points of direct contact. Where cancellous bone is not in contact, the gap will be filled only by being encroached upon by the slow spread of union from the points of contact where it originally started. In other words, *a cut surface of cancellous bone, even with an intact blood supply, does not 'throw out' callus* as does, for instance, the

6

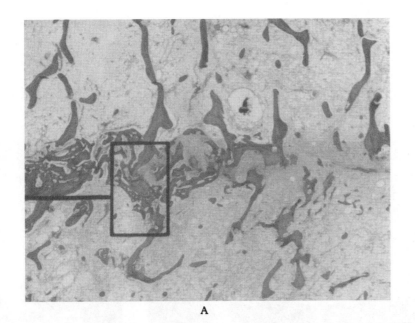

A

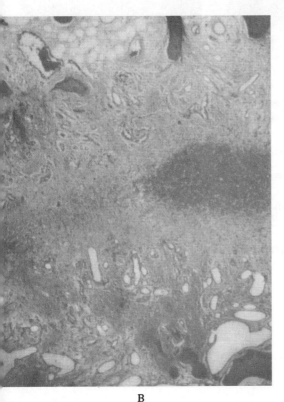

B

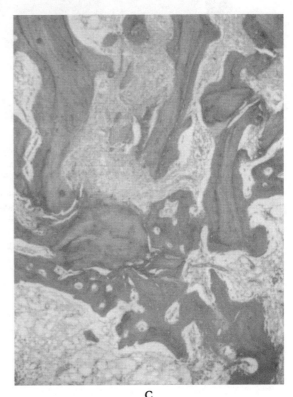

C

Fig. 8

Histology of biopsy taken from same knee fusion to which Fig. 6 and Fig. 7 relate. Four weeks after operation. Clinically solid.

A, Low power showing bridging of woven bone at point of contact (left side), with no bridging across the gap (right side).
B, High power of the gap, showing that the cut ends of the mature trabeculæ have not generated callus.
C, High power of site of union, showing lamellar bone, of original mature trabeculæ, overlaid by the woven bone of newly formed callus (this field has not quite the same vertical orientation as in rectangle of A).

7

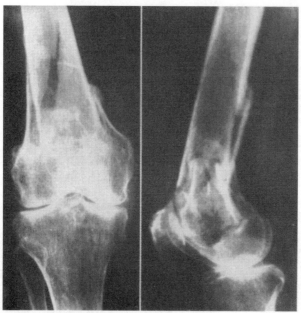

FIG. 9A

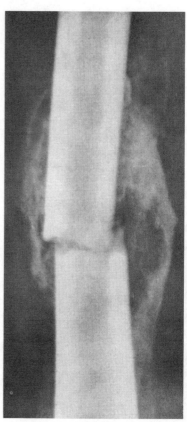

FIG. 9B

Fig. 9A—Fracture in *cancellous* bone at end of a long bone. Note hardly any external periosteal callus though clinically united at three months.

Fig. 9B.—Fracture in *cortical* bone in the centre of a muscle-covered long bone (shaft of femur). Note voluminous ensheathing callus production by periosteum.

Note that periosteal callus springs from surface of bone a short distance from the end of the fragment; this indicates ischæmia of the bone ends.

shaft of the femur. The trabeculæ of cancellous bone adjacent to a blood-filled space will produce the woven bone of callus for a thickness, at the most, only one or two cells deep. I shall emphasise this point repeatedly when describing the union of the shafts of long bones, because I think *the term ' callus ' should be reserved for the voluminous, space-filling, often space-bridging, tissue of woven bone which I believe is generated only in the periosteum (and endosteum) of long bones.*

This difference in the mode of union of fractures in cancellous bone and cortical bone is well illustrated in Figs. 9A and 9B. The total absence of external callus in the fracture through the lower end of the femur (Fig. 9A) was compatible with early union and this patient, aged seventy years, was walking on the leg at three months with 90 degrees range of knee movement, yet radiologically there is no evidence of external callus. By contrast, the external production of 'ensheathing' callus in the fracture through the shaft of the femur is evident (Fig. 9B).

This lack of callus production by cancellous bone explains the tendency to late collapse in the healing of fractures in cancellous bone which have been distracted. Thus after the reduction of a Colles' fracture a hollow cavity is left in the cancellous end of the radius and some degree of spontaneous collapse under conservative treatment is inevitable. The same thing is frequently observed in basal and pertrochanteric fractures of the neck of the femur ; if these have been over-reduced into coxa valga and maintained like this on weight-traction they will often collapse, *even three months later*, when traction is removed—showing that consolidation has been delayed by holding the gap apart (Figs. 10 and 11). The practical application of this observation, if we are to achieve rapid and sound consolidation, therefore indicates the importance of inducing a *controlled degree of collapse* in all fractures involving cancellous bone. If cavities are left inside fractures by over-enthusiastic reduction, there is a danger of *defective consolidation, even in cancellous bone* which in the past has erroneously been regarded as highly osteogenic and incapable of ' delayed union.' A rather extreme example of this is seen in the basal fracture of the neck of the femur already shown in Fig. 1 (p. 2), which occurred in a vigorous sailor of fifty years of age and in whom the metallic internal fixation itself fractured *ten months after the injury.* The patient had evidently been walking on the metallic fixation which, until it fractured by fatigue, was holding apart an unconsolidated fracture in cancellous bone. Had the fracture been allowed initially to collapse into varus, as nature intended, prompt union would have resulted with rapid disappearance of the limp which persists if consolidation is unsound. Another example of this behaviour of cancellous bone is illustrated in Fig. 129, page 164.

In comparing the healing of cancellous bone with cortical bone it is to be noted that in cancellous bone *there appears to be no death of the osteocytes in the cut edges of divided trabeculæ.* This must be because the blood supply is good, and because the large surface area of the trabecular spaces, combined with the relatively thin trabeculæ, keeps the osteocytes nourished by diffusion. The osteocytes deep in the interior of *cortical* bone, on the other hand, cannot receive nourishment by diffusion from the periosteal and endosteal surfaces, and they need the circulation of the Haversian systems to survive. The death of certain areas of osteocytes

9

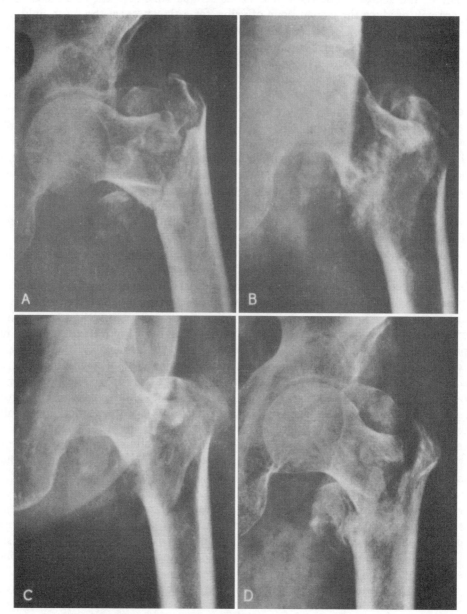

Fig. 10

Pertrochanteric fracture in patient seventy-one years of age treated on continuous traction for three months. A, initial deformity; B, distracted at end of first week; C, traction reduced and position at three months just before final removal of traction; D, position at four months when it appeared clinically united (patient died suddenly of embolism shortly after this film).

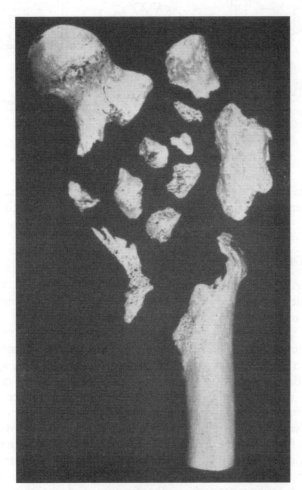

FIG. 11

Same patient as Fig. 10 ; specimen at four months ; very strong fibrous union capable of taking weight ; on digestion with trypsin the fracture was found completely un-united and callus formation minimal. This is probably a common state of affairs at four months if distraction permits the fragments to lie loose and in indefinite contact with each other. Callus did *not* fill up the vacant space left by distraction. Cancellous bone unites only by *contact*, not by throwing out callus to fill spaces.

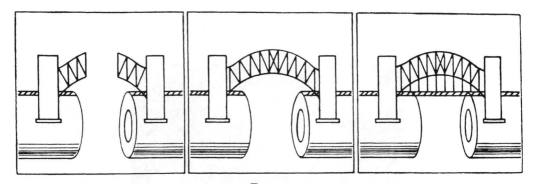

FIG. 12

Hell's Gate Bridge analogy of Urist and Johnson (see text).

in cortical bone would seem to be an inevitable sequel to the cutting of the Haversian systems and the interruption of the longitudinal circulation in the bone ends.

The Union of Cortical Bone

The healing of a fracture through the shaft of human long bones, observed by biopsy studies, has already been described by Urist and Johnson (1943), and I am indebted to this source for the 'two-phase' concept to be described. This two-phase concept is the practical application of the woven bone and lamellar bone sequence mentioned above. Urist and Johnson created the simple but instructive analogy between the healing of the fractured shaft of a long bone and the building of Hell's Gate Bridge (Fig. 12); in the first phase the suspension cables are thrown across the gap (periosteal callus) and in the second phase the permanent roadway is suspended from the cables (the cortical bone of the shaft).

Phase I.—Very soon after a fracture of a long bone, callus (woven bone) appears a short distance from the fractured end of the bone, distributed as a collar encircling the bone and lying in the periosteum between its outer fibrous layer and the surface of the bone. In longitudinal sections this collar of callus [1] is seen as a wedge with the pointed end trailing away from the fracture and the thick end presenting towards the fracture.

It is to be noted that this new bone appears in the periosteum, where a free blood supply is available, and that *the broken end of the bone*, where the longitudinal Haversian circulation is interrupted, *produces no callus whatsoever* (Fig. 13). Callus is also produced on the endosteal aspect of the fracture, where the circulation and endosteal cells are available for osteogenesis, but this does not appear to be such an active source of callus in the human as it is in small animals (probably because bone situated in the axis of the shaft is not mechanically efficient—hence the tubular structure of long bones).

[1] I shall frequently use the term *collar of callus* or *periosteal collar* in this sense in subsequent descriptions.

Under favourable conditions (which we do not yet by any means understand and which constitute the crux of the fracture-healing problem) the collars of periosteal callus bridge the fracture gap by extending through the periphery of the fracture hæmatoma. In some cases callus is apparently able to extend in this way through muscle. This spread of callus from each fragment is preceded by a spindle-celled tissue in which the intercellular spaces become œdematous and in which areas of amorphous intercellular substance appear to condense, to become in some parts islands of hyaline cartilage and in others the woven bone of callus.

This exuberant mass of callus generated by periosteal activity forms the well-known 'plumber's weld' between the fragments. It is often not realised how intense is the cellular activity of the tissue producing this temporary callus. Mitotic figures are seen and the whole mass, especially in bones such as the humerus and femur, often reaches a total diameter three times greater than the diameter of the shaft itself. The whole of this great volume of new tissue is produced in something like three weeks, a degree of activity rivalling that of any sarcoma, and in fact histologically it is not unlike a sarcoma and has occasionally been the cause of serious diagnostic errors. This type of exuberant cellular activity is never seen in the healing of fractures in cancellous bone.

Inside the hollow sphere formed by the invasion of the outer regions of the fracture hæmatoma by callus, the broken bone ends, with their longitudinal circu-

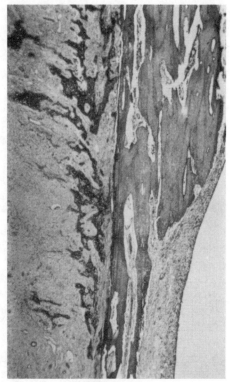

FIG. 13

Callus and cortical fragment from fracture of shaft of femur at four weeks. Note voluminous external *periosteal* callus at left of figure (partly invaded by the woven bone of callus). Note total absence of callus from fractured surface of bone on the right of figure.

lation interrupted, project into the liquefied centre of the fracture hæmatoma and are seen as dead white fragments which to the naked eye appear inert and totally devoid of callus. These features are easily recognised in the specimen illustrated (Fig. 14) from a patient of sixty years of age who died from pulmonary embolus twenty-eight days after a fracture of the shaft of a femur.

The interesting mechanical feature of this phase of 'bridging the gap' is that periosteal callus can cross the gap *even though the fragments are moving in relation to each other*. This bridging seems to be achieved by the fact that the callus extends in the *outer layers* of the hæmatoma, because interstitial movement is less here than it would be in the layers close to the ends of the moving bones. To make an analogy, consider what happens if two sticks are put end to end, to represent a transverse fracture, and the junction is then gripped in the surgeon's closed

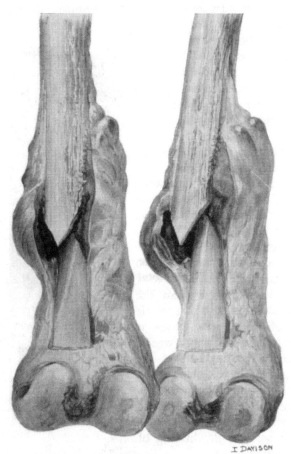

FIG. 14

Artist's drawing of periosteal ensheathing callus of a fractured femur clinically firm twenty-eight days after the injury. Note thickness of callus and the central cavity containing the white, ischæmic bone ends *which themselves are devoid of callus.*

hand (Fig. 15). The sticks can easily be angulated in relation to each other and movement is communicated to the skin on the inside of the closed hand; but the skin on the outside of the hand does not move. It is in this outer stationary zone of the ensheathing callus that the periosteal bone first spreads. Once continuity has been established the sheath of callus starts to thicken and contract down on to the fracture and so immobilises it (Fig. 16). Radiological examples of what is expressed diagrammatically in Fig. 14 will be seen by comparing Fig. 9B, a large hollow callus in the early stage, with Fig. 17 in the later stages. Nature has thus done its own internal fixation (or better still its own bone grafting) of the fracture. This is the stage of ' clinical union ' where function has started to return yet radiologically the fragments are still clearly visible inside the sheath of periosteal callus. Radiologically one would never suspect that inside the sheath of

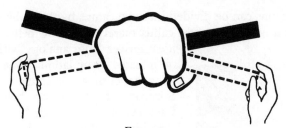

FIG. 15

Analogy of ensheathing callus gripping a fracture even though the fragments are moving slightly. The skin on the exterior of the hand is stationary, but the bones are moving inside the clenched fist.

callus the extreme ends of the fragments are ischæmic, but there is no doubt that this is often the case.

Phase II.—This is the start of the reconstruction of the tubular cortex by the

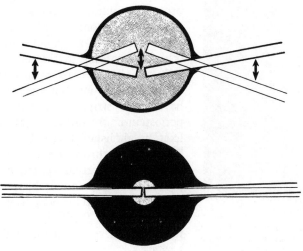

FIG. 16

Scheme to illustrate progressive fixation of moving fragments as ensheathing callus becomes thicker and shrinks on the enclosed fragments.

deposition of lamellar bone, and when it is complete, which takes many months, the ensheathing callus of Phase I will have been completely removed. Lamellar bone cannot be deposited unless there is a solid framework on which it can be deposited. This implies that it can never bridge a gap unless there is a solid scaffold of woven bone already passing across the gap. This is the only phase of fracture repair which necessitates rigid fixation.

The Function of the Periosteum

Fracture surgeons can be divided into two camps by the shibboleth of periosteal callus. One camp sees in profuse callus merely a sign of inefficient union. This idea derives from analogy with the exuberance of infected granulation tissue which we know is made even more exuberant by movement. Surgeons in this camp believe that 'ideal' fracture union should be devoid of ensheathing callus and that it should occur only between the bone ends. They see this absence of periosteal callus after open reduction and rigid internal fixation, and if callus develops after open reduction they suspect that the internal fixation is imperfect and that mobility is evoking periosteal callus.

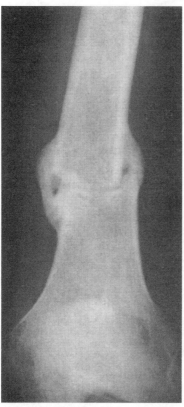

FIG. 17

Compare this illustration with Fig. 9B to see, in actual fact, shrinkage of callus illustrated diagrammatically in Fig. 16. Note persistence of central cavity. Ends of fragments probably still ischæmic though not demonstrable radiologically.

Surgeons of the other camp see in profuse ensheathing callus a highly specialised natural process, a unique process, by which internal fixation is spontaneously achieved between fragments which are moving in relation to each other. According to this concept, ensheathing callus is abolished by open operations, not by the immobilisation but because the bone ends have been stripped of the callus-producing periosteum. According to this opinion, internal fixation abolishes Phase I of normal fracture healing and throws on the surgeon the onus of providing internal fixation as durable as that produced at the end of Phase I until the start of Phase II is well under way. The defective replacement of Phase I, by imperfect internal fixation, will render it impossible for Phase II to start.

Most clinicians who are exponents of internal fixation subconsciously believe that union takes place between the bone ends. But repeated histological examination of the healing of human fractures, reported by many authors, has shown that the ends of cortical bone always show death of osteocytes and that there is never any osteogenic activity from the broken bone surfaces.

The absence of callus between the ends of the bones in a closed, and almost

16

undisplaced, fracture is well illustrated in Fig. 18. The absence of callus between the ends of the bones obviously is not due to any defect of osteogenic potential in the patient, because profuse periosteal callus is bridging the gap in the immediate vicinity of the line of the fracture but separated from it by an appreciable distance. Examples of this pattern of periosteal callus distribution will be discovered very

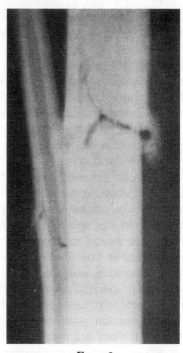

FIG. 18

Unusual amount of periosteal callus for a tibial fracture. There had been minimal displacement in this case. Rapid union.

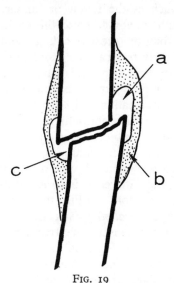

FIG. 19

Illustrating the three essential features of ensheathing callus which can usually be detected in a fracture healing under natural conditions : (a), central cavity inside callus ; (b), callus springing from the periosteum some distance from the end of the bone ; (c), short length of external bone surface, immediately adjacent to the fracture, from which no callus is produced.

frequently once the surgeon starts to examine radiographs with this in mind and the diagram in Fig. 19 emphasises the essential features.

Exuberant Callus and Defective Fixation

The generally accepted opinion that the loosening of internal fixation stimulates the production of periosteal callus, and vice versa, needs careful scrutiny and I doubt the validity of this traditional statement for the following reasons :

1. The production of periosteal new bone after defective internal fixation is *not* callus in what I believe should be the true sense of that word. New periosteal bone generated in the presence of inefficient internal fixation is merely the same thickening of the bone ends which is seen in any pseudarthrosis. It is a *late* phenomenon, not becoming evident until the fracture is at least three or four

months old. Though histologically it is woven bone, and is arising in periosteum (see Fig. 29, p. 28), this is not what I mean by the term *callus*. The ensheathing callus of a normal fracture is visible in the radiograph *very early* (*i.e.*, from three to six *weeks*) and is seen as a cloud or haze standing away some considerable distance from the surface of the bone. This is especially seen in bones such as the femur or humerus which give origin to muscle fibres (Fig. 20A). The total volume of this ensheathing callus after three weeks is many times greater than the greatest enlargement of the bone ends in a pseudarthrosis. This type of early *true* callus I most emphatically maintain is never seen after an open reduction if the bone ends have been stripped of their periosteum.

2. If rigid internal fixation is performed *without stripping the periosteum*, a cloud of *true* callus will develop at the usual time of three to four weeks if the bone is one which normally produces callus. This can frequently be demonstrated in the human subject by inserting an intramedullary nail into a transverse fracture of the shaft of the femur *without disturbing the periosteum*, which can be done if blunt dissection alone is used during the exposure of the bone ends. It is instructive to note the difference in *true* callus production in the two cases illustrated in Figs. 20A and 20B. In Fig. 20A the fixation was rigid and *special care had been taken to avoid periosteal stripping* ; the callus production is profuse and what one would expect in the conservative treatment of a patient of this age (eighteen years). In the second case (Fig. 20B) an assistant did not use special precautions to preserve the periosteum and at the same time he had trouble with the ' jamming ' of an intramedullary nail which had to be cut off because it could not be extracted ; the case was thereafter treated on a Thomas splint. Mobility was present because internal fixation was defective, but this did not stimulate the production of exuberant callus, *even though the patient was only sixteen years of age, when callus production is usually vigorous*. It is to be noted that there is a suspicion of ischæmia of the end of the proximal fragment. There was no clinically recognisable infection.

Those who deny any great importance to the adult periosteum are in part influenced by the insignificant appearance of this tissue if looked for at operation in elderly patients, and in part by the fact that the regeneration of bone after subperiosteal resection is not a particularly noticeable feature in the adult. Similarly, the last echoes still sound of the famous dispute on the function of the periosteum which was settled for the last generation by the weighty opinion of Sir William Macewen in the statement that the periosteum was merely a limiting membrane with negligible osteogenic activity.

That the production of early, voluminous periosteal callus is a purposive mechanism in fracture union (as opposed to an accidental side-effect of movement, not beneficial, and not primarily concerned in fracture repair) must surely be suggested by the enormous histological activity concerned in the growth of periosteal callus. This activity has no counterpart in the repair of any other normal tissue in the body and it can only be compared to a controlled neoplastic growth similar to a sarcoma. In three weeks the volume of ensheathing callus can attain a size three or four times the diameter of the parent bone. This is surely a unique phenomenon with a very definite purpose.

A similar teleological argument is seen in the structure of periosteal callus which obeys mechanical laws. Mechanically the most efficient place in which to use a scanty amount of a relatively weak substance (woven bone) to make a structure rigid, is to place it as far from the axis of movement as possible. This is the principle of 'stressed skin' construction in aircraft and it is the principle extensively used in nature when designing bones as tubular structures.

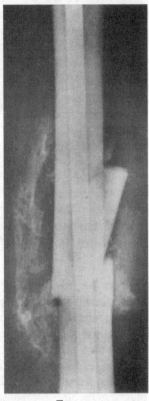

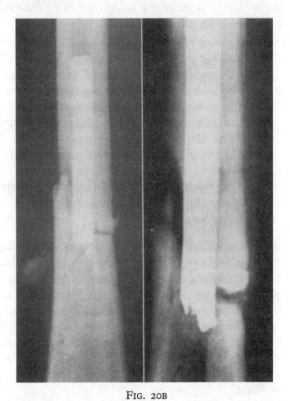

FIG. 20A

True periosteal callus (early and profuse) in youth of eighteen years, six weeks after fracture of shaft of femur. Special care taken not to scrape away periosteum at operation. Fixation rigid.

FIG. 20B

Absence of periosteal callus in youth of sixteen years of age. Fixation was defective. Periosteal surface of the bone had been exposed and cleaned during operation.

The Role of Fixation in Fracture Union

When fractures occur in bones which naturally produce a large volume of ensheathing callus, union will proceed in the presence of movement because the ensheathing callus, when it hardens, produces a natural internal fixation. There are, however, other bones, such as the lower third of the tibia, in which fractures do not produce enough ensheathing callus to ensure internal fixation, and in these it might seem reasonable to imagine that defective ensheathing callus might be compensated by the artificial enhancement of fixation. This is the orthodox argument which is usually accepted without question as a self-evident truth. I believe that a logical examination of this orthodox argument will show that it is by no means as sound as might at first sight appear.

The orthodox argument in favour of the fixation of fractures is that whenever minute bridges of ensheathing callus succeed in jumping the fracture gap they are immediately ruptured by movements of the bone ends. It is assumed that these minute bridges will be ruptured by smaller ranges of movement than would be needed to rupture the bridging of a profuse ensheathing callus. This argument is fallacious for three reasons :

1. It makes the assumption that the gap *has indeed been successfully bridged* even if only by a single minute bridge. It therefore assumes what is the fundamental problem of fracture union—*i.e., how* the first strand of woven bone gets across in the presence of movement.

2. The woven bone of ensheathing callus is almost certainly capable of bending, within certain limits, without being ruptured.

3. When the fragments are *completely immobilised*, as is easily obtained by internal fixation, delayed union is still a frequent occurrence. In other words, the minute bridge of callus, which we assume that faulty immobilisation ruptures, does not hypertrophy even if it is protected from rupture by extreme immobilisation, *for the simple reason that the bridge has never existed.*

The fundamental error in delayed union would seem to be the inability to *start the bridging* of the fracture gap, not the inability to maintain or to augment the first minute strand of callus to get across. The fundamental defect would seem to be the absence of ' callus pathways ' to conduct osseous union from one fragment to the other. There is therefore no logical reason why fixation, *per se*, should facilitate the bridging of a gap if the callus shows no readiness to ' jump the gap ' because no callus pathways are present. There is something in this idea rather analogous to the function of a ' flux ' in soldering metal ; the solder, which can be present in adequate amount, is of no avail if the flux is absent or unsuitable.

An argument advanced in favour of internal fixation is that if rigid fixation can be maintained without mechanical failure for an adequately long period of time all fractures so treated will unite. If the mechanical device fails, by defects of mechanical design in the apparatus at present available, they argue that this does not upset the fundamental premise, and this spurs them on to stronger designs of internal splints. Those who argue in this way are not perturbed by the possibility that the method of fixation may depress osteogenic activity ; they maintain that even if osteogenic activity is depressed the nutrition of the whole limb is improved and joint movement is encouraged, so that when union eventually does occur the result will be better than from conservative treatment.

An element of truth in this last practical argument cannot be denied, but as regards the fundamental nature of osseous union the theory of absolute fixation is specious. A fracture which is ' plate solid ' after good internal fixation can only be revealed as un-united when the apparatus of internal fixation breaks or becomes loose. To illustrate this, consider the case illustrated in Fig. 21.

The patient was a man of thirty-five years with a closed fracture in the midshaft of the femur with slight comminution. An intramedullary nail was inserted one day after the injury but no graft was used (Fig. 21C). The magnitude of the original displacement (Fig. 21A) indicated that delayed union was probable. The radiograph eleven months later is seen in Fig. 21B ; there is very little periosteal callus and callus is ' piling up ' at the fracture line and not flowing across the fracture line as would happen in normal union eleven months after such a fracture, but no definite pseudarthrosis can be diagnosed.

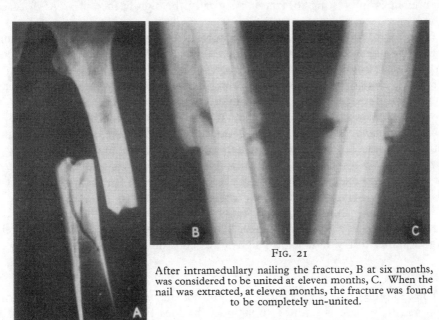

FIG. 21

After intramedullary nailing the fracture, B at six months, was considered to be united at eleven months, C. When the nail was extracted, at eleven months, the fracture was found to be completely un-united.

The radiograph is compatible with union but not proof of union. On clinical tests the fracture was thought to be united and was regarded as an excellent result. Unfortunately the Kuntscher nail was too long and the distal end was threatening to involve the knee joint though causing no symptoms. For this reason it was thought desirable to remove the nail as soon as possible and the decision to do so was made on the clinical evidence of union, hoping that osseous union might be more advanced than the radiograph suggested. At operation the fracture was clearly un-united when the nail was extracted. A second nail, thicker and shorter was easily driven down the track of the first nail and a graft of autogenous iliac bone was laid on the surface of the fibrous union.

The protagonists of internal fixation will say that this nail did not produce absolute fixation. In cases where the intramedullary nail has fractured by fatigue, so demonstrating that the bone is not united,[1] this argument is difficult to deny because the fracture is mobile when it is examined. In the above example, however, it was possible to examine the state of union before extracting the nail ;

[1] Fatigue fracture of a femoral Kuntscher nail has occurred most often in my experience between ten and twelve months after insertion.

the patient possessed a thin thigh which made manual testing quite easy, and with the patient under anæsthesia no detectable motion could be elicited.

This example shows that immobilisation of the fragments of a fracture for eleven months to a degree which is considerably more perfect than is ever possible by conservative means did not enhance the power of union in the fragments.

Fixation and the Speed of Union

In considering whether the role of fixation is fundamental to the union of fractures, it is interesting to examine logically the significance of *speed* in osseous union.

In animals, and even in the human subject, the development of clinical union after a fracture is often an astonishingly rapid process. It is not uncommon to detect clinical union six weeks after fractures of long bones which have been left overriding. Indeed the human tibia, which is notorious for its tendency to delayed union, sometimes can show clinical union in six weeks, even in the adult. Is it not logical to assume therefore that if any factor is fundamental to osseous repair, to enhance this factor should do more than merely eliminate non-union in the end results? If truly fundamental, to enhance fixation should *shorten the average time for clinical union towards the commonly encountered minimum.* If lack of adequate fixation were the sole factor responsible for delayed union of the tibia under conservative treatment, enhancement of the missing factor, as by internal fixation, should produce union so rapidly that it would have been recognised a quarter of a century ago. In practice, internal fixation usually delays the appearance of the radiological signs of osseous union.

Coaptation

I have argued that the essential cause of non-union lies in the failure to bridge a gap and that there is nothing to support the idea that fixation can facilitate the bridging of a gap.

The deduction that coaptation is more important than fixation will be rejected by those who have had the experience of delayed union after internal fixation *when there has been perfect coaptation.* The crux of the matter must surely lie in the *vitality of the bone ends* which have been accurately coapted. If these bone ends have had their blood supply completely interrupted, and their capacity to produce ensheathing callus destroyed by the periosteal covering having been stripped from the edges of the fracture, the perfection of coaptation, judged radiologically, is of no significance. In this case two utterly inert fragments have been coapted. This is proved by the experience reported in relation to Fig. 21.

Ischæmia of Bone Ends Increased by Surgery

Examples of the devitalisation of bone fragments by operative intervention on fractures are illustrated in the following case histories:

1. Fig. 22 is a gross example of the inhibition of callus formation at the actual site of the fracture produced by operative exposure. The failure of callus to 'jump

the gap' between the bone ends is astonishing in view of the fact that the power to produce callus must have been considerable since it could successfully take such a devious pathway. This must surely indicate that the ends of the fragments were dead and ischæmic even though there is no radiological evidence of this.

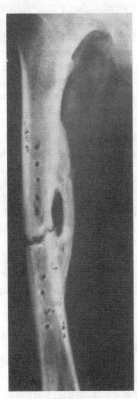

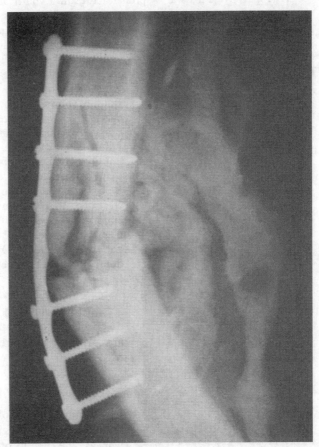

FIG. 22

Example 1 (see text).

FIG. 23

Showing absence of callus between ends of the bone, after internal fixation, even in a case possessing a strong potential for callus production.

2. A similar circuitous method by which callus has by-passed a fracture is illustrated in Fig. 23. There is obviously no lack of osteogenic potential in this patient, but none of it has been revealed between the bone ends. This example indicates in an exaggerated way the usual process of union after the operative treatment of fractures.

3. Fig. 24 illustrates an oblique fracture of the tibia in a man of sixty-two years of age treated by the insertion of two transverse screws and the application of a plaster cast. Four months later the fracture was mobile and it was apparent that the screws had cut out. The fracture was re-operated on to apply bone grafts of autogenous iliac bone, and it was immediately obvious that the proximal fragment of the tibia was dead and white. A biopsy was taken and the site of its removal is visible in the radiograph. Histologically there was no evidence of infection. There would seem to be no doubt that

the initial operative intervention destroyed any osteogenic potential in this fracture and union would probably have been uneventful if the case had been treated conservatively.

4. (Fig. 25.) This was a spiral fracture in a youth of twenty, which was treated by two transverse screws. The technical details of the operation were beyond criticism and the reduction was such that the fracture line was invisible in the post-operative film. Eleven weeks after the operation the youth fell over a raised curb, re-fracturing his leg while still in a long leg plaster. X-ray of the displaced fracture shows that the osteosynthesis has come apart exactly as it was before the operation and that this is due to breaking of one screw and avulsion of the other. It is therefore reasonable to deduce that little or no osseous union was present at eleven weeks, and that the fracture was dependent only on the screws. By contrast, I am quite certain that under conservative treatment it would have been impossible to move a spiral fracture of this kind eleven weeks after injury if, for example, a remanipulation for mal-position had been needed. Operative interference has thus depressed the osteogenic activity of a very simple fracture.

Further examples extending the thesis of the ill-effects of open operation on callus formation are given in Chapter XV on fractures of the tibia.

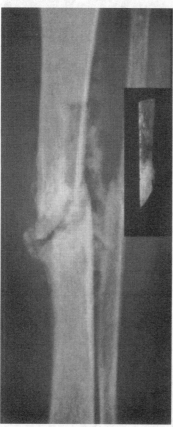

FIG. 24

Inset is biopsy specimen reproduced to same scale as radiograph and site in proximal fragment from which it was removed is visible. Note the dead white end adjacent to fracture. Two transverse screws through an oblique fracture destroy more bone than one screw. Meddlesome surgery.

Circumferential Wiring

The evil effects of a circumferential suture of bone have been recognised ever since the 1914-18 war as the result of experience with Parham's band. There is still a tendency to revive the use of the circumferential suture of wire stimulated by the invention of attractive wire-tightening gadgets. Results, typical of the evil effects of this method, are illustrated in Figs 26 and 27. This result can be explained by the fact that :

1. Periosteal stripping has suppressed ensheathing callus.
2. The metal encirclement presents a permanent barrier to bridging by collars of periosteal callus.

Biologically and mechanically this method is the worst of any method of internal fixation. It is an even more pernicious way of killing part of a long bone than by sandwiching it between two large metal plates ; in the latter there is at least

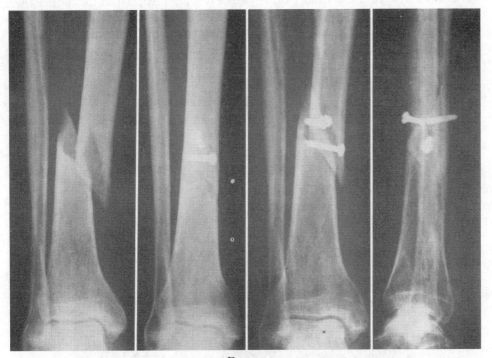

FIG. 25

Anatomical reduction, but the anatomically reduced ends have been devitalised by operation. Complete re-fracture eleven weeks later. This spiral fracture could have been treated better conservatively.

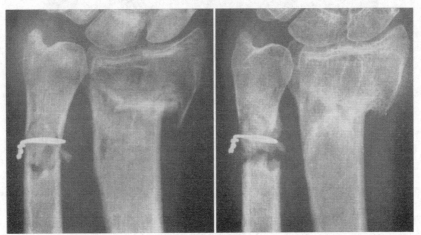

FIG. 26

Destruction of bone by 'encirclage' (see text).

good fixation, even if the vitality of the bones is imperilled, but in the former there is neither fixation nor vitality. Some of the evil of circumferential wiring can be diminished by drilling a hole through both fragments and encircling only half of the circumference of the fracture, but the fixation is not as good even as that

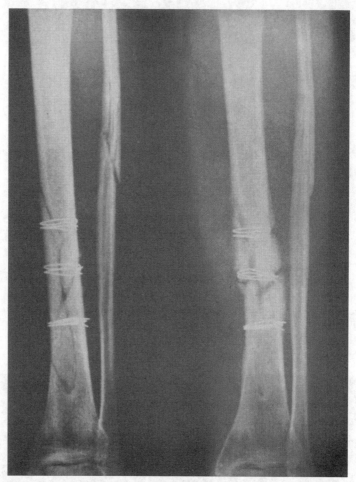

FIG. 27

Evil effects of multiple encirclage. There was no clinical evidence of infection in this case. The illustration on the left was six weeks after the operation ; on the right are the appearances nine months later.

obtained by a transverse screw in oblique fractures, which I have criticised elsewhere.

When one considers the diagram in Fig. 28 the disastrous effect of ' encirclage ' on an oblique fracture is fairly obvious. The fact that many cases are still able to unite after this operation is no tribute to the method—it merely indicates that the bones in such cases had remarkable powers for uniting *in spite of* the method.

Fracture Union as a Local Phenomenon

No account of the phenomenon of fracture union is complete without a reference to the possible existence of systemic factors. Every patient with delayed union wants reassurance that his diet is adequate and whether or not he should take calcium and vitamins. There are a number of clinical facts indicating that in delayed union systemic factors are of negligible importance and that local factors are all-important :

1. Old people, and patients with debilitating disease, often have less trouble with the union of fractures than do strong healthy men. This is particularly the case in the tibia, and it is possible that this can be explained by the fact that when cortical bone becomes porotic it is because of the enlargement of its Haversian canals, and therefore it has an exceptionally good blood supply ; the dense bone

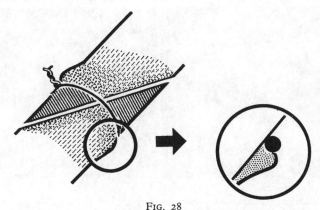

Fig. 28

Diagram showing the idea that encirclage can devitalise bone fragments and also prevent the extension of periosteal callus.

of the athletic young adult, on the other hand, has small Haversian canals because they are encroached on by the much greater amount of inert bone mineral needed for the function of weight-bearing.

2. When multiple fractures occur in the same patient, one of these, such as the shaft of a femur, may unite rapidly whereas another, such as the shaft of the tibia, may show delay in union, and even progress to true non-union.

3. In double fracture of the same bone, one fracture almost invariably unites quickly while the other is delayed, or even develops into non-union.

4. A close inspection of any established non-union reveals that there is considerable new bone formation, as shown by the piling up of subperiosteal bone on each side of the fracture gap, which produces considerable thickening of the bone ends. It is evident that the essential failure of union is the failure to bridge the gap, *not the failure to generate bone*. This is well demonstrated in Fig. 29 where the increased width of the shaft of a metacarpal in the presence of non-union can be compared with the width of the bone at the time of the fracture.

27

Sepsis and the Periosteum

In any discussion on the operative treatment of fractures the serious effects of sepsis cannot be ignored. Why should bones be more susceptible to infection than most other connective tissues ? Again, it is possible that the answer is to be found in the function of the periosteum. The vitality of the surface of a bone resides in its periosteal blood supply, and with its clothing of periosteum preserved intact a bone possesses very high resistance to infection, even if surrounded by pus on all sides. Inflamed periosteum reacts by producing new bone which is seen to an extreme degree in the 'involucrum' of hæmatogenous osteomyelitis. When, however, the periosteum is stripped from the underlying bone, as in performing the internal fixation of a fracture, the vitality of the surface of the bare bone is abolished and the physical conditions are thus highly favourable for

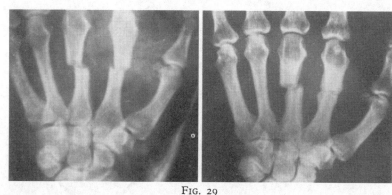

FIG. 29

Delayed union. Compare the diameter of fragments immediately after fracture and four months later. Plentiful production of callus but essential error is *failure of callus to bridge the gap.*

the continuation of sepsis—and even more so if metallic foreign bodies are present. One cannot help thinking that many cases of delayed union after internal fixation may be the result of deep infection which has been masked, and which has eventually subsided, under the influence of antibiotics (*i.e.*, Fig. 27 is compatible with this possibility though no clinical evidence of infection was present).

An instructive lesson can be learned from inspecting the 'coronet' or 'ring' sequestrum which used to be a common occurrence in infected amputation stumps with the old surgeons. It is probable that the coronet sequestrum reveals the volume of bone rendered avascular by the division of the longitudinal circulation at the time of section and by the periosteal stripping at the site chosen for sawing the bone. Without sepsis this volume of bone would be ischæmic but would become reincorporated without ever becoming recognisable radiographically ; but the addition of infection will kill the ischæmic zone completely and the adjacent bone will form a line of demarcation and a radiological sequestrum will then be revealed. It is but a short cry from this example to that of an infected fracture, because an amputation is nothing more than the proximal half of a compound fracture. The two illustrations (Figs. 30 and 31) illustrate the 'ring'

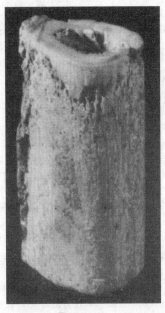

FIG. 30

' Ring' sequestrum of femur from septic amputation stump, discovered in John Hunter's Collection, Royal College of Surgeons of England. Sepsis has demarcated zone of ischæmia produced by interruption of the longitudinal circulation. (*By courtesy of the Curator, Dr Proger.*)

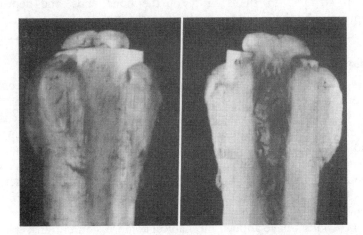

FIG. 31

Septic amputation stump dissected and prepared by John Hunter (collection of Royal College of Surgeons of England) to show fibro-cartilaginous callus. Note ischæmic end of bone and how external callus does not reach end of bone. *No callus produced by the end of the bone itself.* (*By courtesy of the Curator, Dr Proger.*)

29

sequestra encountered in amputation stumps when infection has rendered irreversible the area of ischæmia produced in the bone end by section of the longitudinal Haversian systems by the saw. Had these amputation stumps been aseptic these ring sequestra would have been reincorporated. These illustrations show vividly the futility of expecting the ends of cortical bone to join when they are coapted or compressed together. Union in this case could only be by the development of an ensheathing callus. It is interesting to observe that the specimen in Fig. 31 shows how the ensheathing callus heaps up round the bone end but fails to project beyond the end of the bone and even falls short by the distance the cortex is ischæmic. It is fascinating to record that these two specimens are from John Hunter's own collection and that they are nearly two hundred years old. They were found and photographed for me by Dr Proger, Curator of the Hunterian Collection, and I am deeply indebted to him and the Royal College of Surgeons for permission to make use of these historic exhibits.

Anatomical Explanation of Ischæmia of Bone Ends

The anatomical explanation of local ischæmia affecting the ends of a broken long bone is illustrated diagrammatically in Fig. 32, A and B. The longitudinal arrangement of the blood vessels inside the Haversian systems is shown and the manner in which they connect with each other by transverse anastomoses. The blood vessels of the periosteum reinforce this longitudinal circulation through similar transverse channels, as do also the medullary vessels on the endosteal aspect. When the bone is severed a continuous circulation of blood inevitably must stop in those parts of the divided Haversian canals which lie between the broken surface and the nearest subjacent transverse anastomosis. When the periosteum is stripped in the vicinity of the bone ends, the deprivation of blood supply to the bone ends is significantly increased and corresponds to the 'ring' sequestra illustrated in Figs. 30 and 31. (John Hunter's specimens.)

Compression in the Union of Fractures

There is evidence that powerful mechanical compression, acting continuously for three to four weeks, has a beneficial action on the union of *cancellous* bone (Charnley, 1953), but I am not convinced that there is good evidence that compression stimulates the union of fractures in *cortical* bone. The interruption of the longitudinal circulation in the ends of long bones, caused by the fracture inter-rupting Haversian systems, is in itself enough to explain the futility of compressing together bone ends which are composed of little more than an inert mineral substance. The broken ends of the cortex are the only inert surfaces in a fracture where everywhere else is a hive of cellular activity.

On two occasions I have applied mechanical compression to transverse fractures of the tibia by transfixing the bones above and below the fracture with Steinmann nails and applying compression clamps as in compression arthrodesis of the knee. After six weeks of compression there was no evidence of clinical union. After six weeks of compression in cancellous bone clinical union would be present in three cases out of four.

Various writers have reported successful union following the application of compression to *delayed union* and even to *non-union* in fractured long bones. That osseous union might be precipitated by this means is consistent with general experience that weight-bearing is beneficial *in the later stages* of fracture treatment, but experience has not shown weight-bearing to be beneficial in the early stages of treatment.

Eggers (1949) found evidence of increased osteogenic activity in pressure experiments on the rat's skull, but it was difficult to dissociate these results from

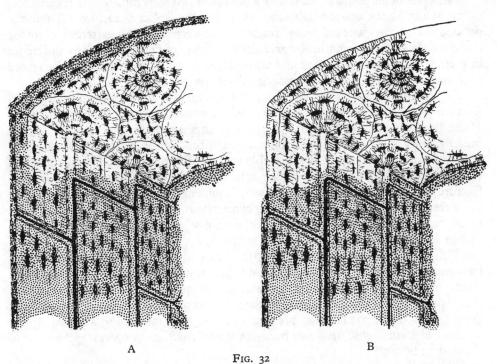

A   B

FIG. 32

Diagram of Haversian systems in the cortex of the divided end of a long bone.   The nutrition of the divided end of the bone is indicated, A, when the periosteum is intact and B, when the periosteum has been stripped for some distance near the end of the bone.   (*Adapted from Fig. 138, Ham, 'Histology,' 1950, J. B. Lippincott.*)

the mere effects of 'contact' without compression. Eggers found destructive changes when the 'contact-compression factor' was excessive. Friedenberg and French (1952), using an ingenious spring compression device on the ulna of the dog, found evidence of good union when forces not more than 30 lb. were used, but above this union was impeded; their technique, though ingenious, would seem to me to prejudice the circulation of the experimental fracture.

Magnitude of Initial Displacement in Relation to Union

Of all the factors which influence the speed of union of a fracture through the shaft of a long bone probably the most important relates to the magnitude of the initial displacement. If we consider the particular case of a fracture in the shaft of the tibia, no one will dispute the general statement that a fracture with only slight displacement will unite rapidly after the most perfunctory treatment, even though the tibia is a bone notoriously prone to delayed union. On the other hand, a fracture of the tibia with gross initial displacement will often fail to unite even though it may be reduced perfectly; indeed, so perfectly that the radiological appearance may be superior to the previous example in which the initial slight displacement is accepted without reduction.

The bone of an undisplaced fracture is broken just as completely as regards loss of continuity of the osseous substance as a grossly displaced fracture. There are no degrees in the state of being fractured between the two extremes of being *broken* or *not broken* except in the greenstick fracture of childhood. Any difference in the rate of union of displaced and undisplaced fractures must therefore be traced to differences in the state of the associated soft parts.

An argument which might challenge this statement is the occasional undisplaced fracture which fails to unite. This is most commonly seen in oblique fractures of the tibia with an intact fibula. I can only suggest that in this type of case the initial radiograph does not reveal the true magnitude of the displacement sustained at the moment of violence. It is possible that the elasticity of the fibula, combined with the flexibility of the tibio-fibular articulations, could protect the fibula from fracture while the tibial fragments were momentarily separated by a distance great enough to tear all local soft tissue connections. It is often forgotten that the initial radiograph of any fracture is made after first-aid workers have ' straightened up ' gross external deformities existing at the site of the accident.

This certainly can happen in Pott's fractures of the ankle; I have seen this fracture diagnosed as ' undisplaced ' on the initial radiograph, and for this reason entrusted to an inexperienced assistant to apply a plaster, with the result that ' spontaneous ' displacement has been discovered later. This is explained by gross tearing of soft parts being present, due to gross initial displacement at the moment of injury which has not been suspected from the innocent appearance of the first radiograph.

The deduction which I think we can reasonably make from this is that the ' bridge ' or ' callus pathway ' which conducts periosteal callus from one fragment to another must lie in the soft tissues investing the fragments. In the case of the tibia an intact connection of both fragments to the interosseous membrane is probably the deciding factor because it is at the site of attachment of the interosseous ligament that callus most often is first seen to bridge the tibial fracture.

This conception of the role of the soft tissues in conducting periosteal callus across a fracture is particularly important in those bones which do not possess the ability to throw out profuse periosteal callus and less important in those muscle-covered bones such as the femur, humerus, and shaft of fibula, which tend to produce a voluminous investing callus. This *fatalistic concept of delayed union as a function of soft-part damage* is expressed diagrammatically in Fig. 33.

Traction and Distraction in the Treatment of Fractures

If we accept the idea that the capacity for rapid union, or for delayed union, is established by the amount of damage to soft parts at the time of injury, arguments condemning the use of continuous traction in the treatment of fractures need to be re-examined. It has been customary to condemn weight-traction because of the danger of causing 'distraction.' A fracture which initially was grossly displaced, associated therefore with extensive tearing of the soft parts, would still suffer from delayed union even if accurate coaptation were obtained without traction.

The two previous editions of this book were dominated by the fear of distraction, and for this reason fixed traction was advocated in preference to all forms of weight-traction. I am now convinced that much of the harm

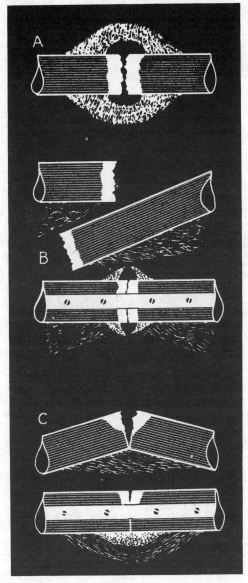

Fig. 33—The fatalistic concept of initial displacement in relation to soft-tissue damage and to osseous union: the preservation, or destruction, of the 'callus pathway' between the fragments.

A, Successful union in that type of bone which is capable of generating profuse periosteal callus. The ischæmic bone ends, even if reduced end to end, do not impede the bridging of callus in this type of case.

B, Fracture with gross initial displacement *in a bone incapable of generating profuse periosteal callus*. End-to-end contact puts the collars of periosteal callus out of reach of each other. No intact soft-part bridge exists as a callus pathway. It is possible that union might have occurred if the fracture had been left undisturbed in this position with overriding and full displacement.

C, Successful union *in a bone incapable of generating profuse periosteal callus*, because minimal displacement preserved a soft-part bridge and hence a callus pathway on the concave side of the fracture.

NOTE.—Open reduction and internal fixation was unnecessary in C; open reduction and internal fixation in B still might not eliminate the necessity for a bone graft.

FIG. 33

which originally was attributed to weight-traction ought to be transferred to the rupture of the pathways which conduct osseous union between the fragments.

We have heard a great deal in the last few years about the harmful effects of

33

distraction in delaying osseous union without considering instances where union has occurred in the presence of distraction. The following case illustrates this point in an exaggerated degree :

The patient (Fig. 34) was eighteen years of age, and a leg-lengthening operation had been performed two years previously, using a long Z-section of the shaft of the femur. The operation succeeded in achieving an elongation of $2\frac{1}{2}$ inches but was followed by slow consolidation. This slow consolidation, without the appearance of periosteal callus, I attributed to extensive periosteal stripping of the femur at the line of operation. While in a walking caliper splint the femur re-fractured three times because the attenuated part of the bone did not show any tendency to hypertrophy. Each of the re-fractures was accompanied by the production of good periosteal callus, which I interpreted as indicating that by this time a new periosteum had formed. All three re-fractures took place while the patient was wearing the caliper splint, so that extensive tearing of soft parts was not to be expected. When the third fracture occurred it was treated by weight-traction which was deliberately excessive and distraction of 1 inch occurred. Callus bridged this gap and the limb was clinically united in three months.

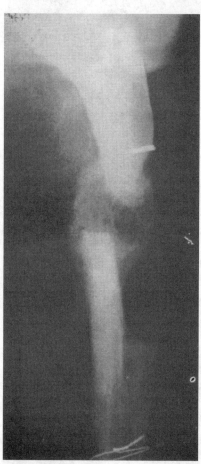

FIG. 34

Showing that the distraction of bone fragments is not in itself the cause of failure to produce callus.

This example is unusual as regards the common behaviour of callus in the healing of a fracture of the femur, but it is customary in the process of leg-lengthening in young patients. It illustrates that distraction by itself is not the sole cause of the failure of callus to bridge a gap. In this example I suggest that the soft parts were still in continuity across the gap and that they were stretched by the traction without being ruptured.

If distraction occurs, using ordinary amounts of traction force, it indicates that severe soft-tissue damage was sustained at the time of the injury and it is a warning that the fracture is likely to suffer delayed union no matter what form of initial treatment is adopted. There is no excuse for tolerating the distraction of fractures, but there is no need to condemn weight-traction as a principle if distraction is avoided. Weight-traction renders a patient much more comfortable than is possible

34

on fixed traction, and for this reason I am now adding balanced traction to methods which originally were designed strictly to avoid continuous traction.

Fibrous Septa as the Callus Pathway

My belief that callus spreads from one fragment to another via the interosseous membrane is illustrated by the example in Fig. 35, where the initial displacement is seen on the left and the appearance six months later is on the right. In this

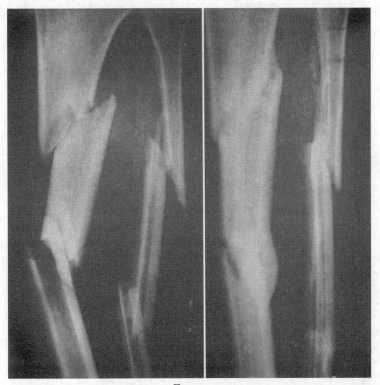

FIG. 35
Illustrating the ' callus pathway ' in the intact tissues on the side of the distal fracture which was concave in the original deformity.

comminuted fracture of the tibia the interest centres round the distal tibial fracture. The concave side of the deformity (*i.e.*, the side on which the soft parts are least torn) is the side of the interosseous septum. The radiograph at six months has been made with an oblique orientation to show the full width of the interosseous space which is not revealed in routine anteroposterior and lateral views. It will be seen that the callus has bridged the fracture in the attachment of the interosseous septum, and that there is no callus on the opposite side of the bone. A similar state of affairs in seen in Fig. 158, page 206.

The function of fibrous tissue in offering a pathway for callus to bridge a fracture is suggested in the examples shown in Figs. 22, 23, 35, and 158 ; if the

35

intermuscular septa arising from the linea aspera of the femur were elevated during the operation for plating they would occupy the position of the bridge of callus in these illustrations.

Primary Bone Grafting in the Treatment of Fractures

If we accept the idea that the delayed union of fractures in cortical bone is decided at the time of the injury by the extent of the tearing of ' callus-pathways,' the immediate use of bone grafts might seem a logical way of establishing a callus-pathway across the ' physiological gap ' which can exist between bone ends which are in perfect anatomical coaptation. We must ask ourselves whether primary bone grafting is quite such a logical procedure as it may appear on first consideration.

I have never been able to satisfy myself that a bone graft in a fresh fracture is any different from a fragment of the fracture itself. A bone graft, being totally ischæmic, will be even more ischæmic than the comminuted fragments already present in the fracture because many of these will possess some vascular connections. A suggestion of this possibility, which I have observed on several occasions, is indicated by the two following case histories :

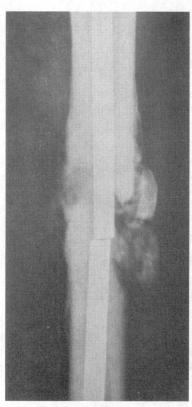

FIG. 36

Failure of autogenous iliac bone-graft to induce union of a fracture when inserted at the time of the primary operation. Non-union was revealed ten months later when the intramedullary nail fractured by fatigue.

Case 1. The patient was a man of fifty years of age with comminuted fracture of the midshaft of the femur, with gross initial displacement, which was treated by open exposure of the fragments and insertion of a Kuntscher nail. The surgeon performing the operation felt he could improve the situation by replacing the loose comminuted fragments of dense cortical bone by slices of autogenous spongiosa of iliac bone because these might fuse into the fracture quicker than cortical bone (Fig. 36). In due course clinical union was considered to be safe and the patient was permitted to take full weight on the limb. Sudden pain was experienced ten months after the injury and fatigue fracture of the nail was discovered, with return of mobility in the fracture, and with clear radiological evidence that the grafted fragments of cancellous bone had not incorporated into the fracture.

Case 2. This was a patient of twenty-four years of age (Fig. 37) who was operated on nine days after the fracture. A four-hole plate was applied, augmented with chips of fresh autogenous iliac bone. Rigid fixation was obtained but because the plate was short

36

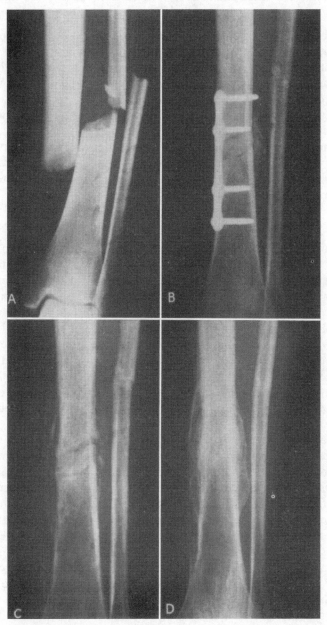

FIG. 37

Autogenous iliac bone-graft, seen on lateral aspect of fracture, B, applied at time of primary operation for plating the tibia. Three months later fracture was un-united and mobile. Appearances three months after application of a second iliac graft and removal of loose plate, C, and appearances one year later, D.

37

a long leg plaster was applied in addition. Three months later, when the second plaster was removed, the fracture had become mobile.

It is my belief that an autogenous graft of cancellous bone is incorporated into a fracture with most uniform success when a delay of several weeks has elapsed between the fracture and the operation. By that time the ends of the bones, and the periosteum, have achieved maximum vascularity and the volume of cortical bone rendered ischæmic at the time of the fracture is at a minimum. Sandwiched between a hyperæmic periosteum and the denuded surface of hyperæmic bone, the bone graft has an optimal chance of incorporation (page 248). If inserted when the fracture is fresh the graft merely denudes the fracture of more periosteum, which increases the volume of ischæmic bone in the fracture, and in some cases the fragments of graft become invested in fibrous tissue and fail to incorporate in the fracture.

Blood Supply and Fracture Repair

Throughout this review of the factors which influence the healing of fractures I have tried to show that mechanical elements are of secondary importance to biological factors. In the treatment of a fresh fracture we can control only the secondary factors, such as accurate reduction and rigid fixation. The full deployment of biological factors in the repair of a fracture depends on augmentation of existing blood supply at the fracture site. The augmentation of blood supply is a process which takes time ; it proceeds at a rate determined by the living tissues in response to the stimulus of fracture. Operative interference at the fracture site can never enhance this process of increasing vascularisation and only too often operative interference isolates the bone fragments from their original blood supply and puts them in a position where the stimulus to hyperæmia cannot take effect.

Cancellous bone usually has a profuse supply of blood and therefore the mechanical factors of accurate reduction and rigid fixation (enhanced by the addition of compression) can be guaranteed to secure union in about four weeks (as judged in arthrodesis of the knee clinically and by the histology of biopsy specimens). When both fragments of a fracture possess an intact supply of blood, both can participate actively in the process of union, and I hold the view that in these circumstances union can take place in the presence of a slight ' hinge ' movement. In fractures where one of the fragments has been deprived of its supply of blood, as in sub-capital fractures of the neck of the femur, the only factors available to encourage union are mechanical. In this special instance we are dealing with conditions which are the same as in bone grafting. When one fragment is ischæmic the ' host ' bone has to revascularise the ischæmic fragment before it can become incorporated, and to do this close apposition and rigid fixation are absolutely necessary. One can summarise these ideas thus :

1. If both fragments are alive, rigid immobilisation is not essential for union.
2. If one fragment is ischæmic, rigid immobilisation is essential for union.
3. If both fragments are ischæmic, rigid immobilisation is futile.

It is when we consider the treatment of fractures in cortical bone (as in the shafts of long bones) that the mechanical elements in treatment are of secondary importance. In cortical bone the supply of blood to the ends of a bone fragment in a fresh fracture is restricted by the small calibre of the Haversian canals which traverse the dense mass of ivory bone. At the moment when a fracture of cortical bone is sustained the proportion of living elements, which ultimately are responsible for the healing of the fracture, is small when compared with the proportion of inert mineral matter which is responsible for the strength of the tubular bone. The density of the ivory bone is an obstacle to repair, but in the course of normal fracture healing the vascular channels enlarge and the dense cortical bone becomes permeated with enlarged vascular channels. Until the cortical bone has become porous there seems no hope of it being able to participate in osseous union. If the ends of the bones are stripped of periosteum by open operation the ability of the Haversian canals to enlarge is seriously impeded and the ends of the bones remain dense long after adjacent parts with intact vascular connections have become porous (Fig. 24, p. 24). Thoughts like this encourage the idea of delay before engaging in the operative treatment of fractures (see p. 41).

Conservative versus Operative Treatment

In discussing the pros and cons of the operative treatment of fractures I shall defer the obvious argument of operative sepsis to the chapter on fractures of the tibia, because it is here that infection is most likely, the tibia being a subcutaneous bone and very frequently compound.

I shall here confine attention to matters which I think are just as important as sepsis, though less obvious, and will consider these under two headings : (1) the harmful effects of operative treatment and (2) the harmful effects of conservative treatment.

The *harmful effects of operative treatment* stem from the depression of osteogenic activity in the fragments of a fracture. Operative exposure increases the volume of ischæmic bone which is always present, even if only in small amount, in any fracture of cortical bone. The extent of this sequel to operation is commonly overlooked because early ischæmia in long bones is not detectable in radiographs. Even in fractures of the femoral neck where ischæmia of the femoral head is anticipated, we know that extreme ischæmia can be present for more than one year without definite radiological evidence. Urist, Mazet, and McLean (1954) investigated operative and conservative treatment in 100 successfully united tibiæ and in eighty-five cases of non-union in the tibia, and I cannot do better than quote extracts which summarise their views. Every surgeon would do well to ponder these statements before embarking on open treatment :

> ' The effect of open operations on fresh fractures is to increase the volume of damaged bone which has to be absorbed and replaced before the fracture can unite and permit full weight-bearing.'

> ' Comminuted fractures of the human adult tibia should be considered non-operable because the trauma added by surgery exceeds the normal capacity for bone regeneration in this area of the skeleton.'

'In fractures with contact between the bone ends, internal fixation has either no effect or no adverse effect on the healing time. It is never a stimulus to bone repair.'

'If a fracture is short and oblique rather than long and spiral and if two or three screws are inserted in order to achieve strong fixation there will frequently be enough necrosis of the bone around the metal to cause disintegration of the entire area of the fracture.'

'The very good results in the majority of non-comminuted fractures could be used as evidence in favour of internal fixation, but the argument is weakened by comparison with the equally good results in matched fractures treated by closed methods.'

'Open reduction and internal fixation of extensively comminuted fractures always prolongs healing and never encourages it.'

The *harmful effects of conservative treatment* of fractures of the shafts of long bones all stem from delayed union and are all related to residual deformity and stiffness of joints.

In both operative and conservative methods of primary treatment we must take into consideration the complications of bone grafting operations if these become necessary as secondary measures.

In comparing the harmful effects of conservative and operative methods it is interesting to consider the three following propositions : (1) that operative treatment is potentially harmful to all fractures,[1] but conservative treatment is harmful only to a few ; (2) that the few fractures which are harmed by conservative treatment would have been less harmed had they been operated ; (3) that the failures of operative and of conservative methods are not equally capable of being salvaged by secondary procedures. It is this last which is the critical point.

Reviewing fractures of the shafts of the long bones in accordance with ideas suggested by the foregoing propositions, I have come to the conclusion that only in two sites are the failures of conservative treatment worse than the failures of operative treatment ; these are (1) middle and upper thirds of the femur (*not* the lower third) and (2) shafts of the radius and ulna.

In the upper half of the shaft of the femur the result of delayed consolidation under conservative treatment is invariably late deformity, because conservative methods, if they have to be used for weeks on end, eventually fail to control alignment in fractures at, or above, the midshaft. To apply a bone graft to a femur in the presence of late angulation and mal-alignment is a formidable procedure. The only method of internal fixation which I consider justifiable when grafting the shaft of the femur is an intramedullary nail, and in order to insert this it is necessary to break down the fracture and expose the medullary canal. If this major procedure is to be done without a delay of many months it will have to be done through tissues which are indurated and slightly œdematous ; this renders the wound prone to operative sepsis and more so if the operating time is prolonged by unforeseen technical difficulties. If, on the other hand, the original

---

[1] I am considering fractures of the shafts of long bones. I do not, of course, include fractures in such bones as the patella, olecranon, and neck of femur where conservative treatment is obviously futile.

fracture has been treated by a Kuntscher nail, and if delayed consolidation has later become evident, the introduction of a subperiosteal graft of iliac bone is a procedure of the utmost simplicity and safety, because it can be postponed until the patient has a fully mobile knee and healthy soft tissues.

The same argument applies to the conservative treatment of fractures of both bones of the forearm : delayed consolidation after conservative treatment is invariably associated with malposition of the radial and ulnar fragments and bone grafting is a formidable procedure necessitating realignment of the fractures in tissues which are often slightly œdematous. If both radius and ulna have to be grafted there is often the special difficulty of closing the skin wounds without tension. On the other hand, if the fractures of the radius and ulna had originally been plated the insertion of subperiosteal grafts of iliac bone by the Phemister technique would have been a relatively minor and safe procedure because it could be carried out through soft tissues which were more or less completely rehabilitated.

This argument in favour of operative treatment (that it facilitates subsequent bone grafting should this become necessary) does not apply with the same force to those fractures where satisfactory alignment can be held by conservative methods. The fractures of long bones which can be held in adequate alignment by conservative treatment are the tibia, the lower third of the femur, and the humerus.

To appreciate fully the argument that the form of the initial treatment of a fresh fracture must be assessed in relation to it facilitating the performance of a bone graft if this should become necessary at a later date, it is necessary to mention the type of bone graft envisaged. The greatest advance in fracture treatment in this century has come from improvements in the technique of bone grafting and not from improvements in the technique of handling the fresh fracture. The type of bone graft which I believe has revolutionised the treatment of fractures is the application of slices of autogenous iliac bone to the surface of the delayed union without disturbing the tissue between the ends of the bones. We owe to Phemister (1947) the first full account of how this simple procedure induces the fibrous union to convert to bone. So important do I consider this technique that I have devoted considerable space to describing how I believe it is best carried out in relation to fractures of the tibia (p. 248).

Delayed Operations on Fractures

When balancing the indications for conservative and operative treatment in a particular clinical problem, there are occasions when the surgeon may feel that if he is to operate he must do so urgently if he is to get a good result. This idea makes him unwilling to try conservative treatment lest he should be driven to open reduction after a delay which might prejudice the result. The phrase ' the timing of the fracture healing process ' has often been bandied about but no definite facts have been adduced and there is a general tendency to recommend early intervention.

In fractures of the shaft of the tibia, if open operation is to be undertaken, it certainly is a matter of considerable urgency because the overlying skin becomes œdematous and unfavourable for surgery in twenty-four to forty-eight hours.

In sites where adequate soft parts cover the fracture and the dangers associated with a subcutaneous bone like the tibia do not exist, there is much to be said for delay before operation. J. E. M. Smith (1959) investigated the results of early and late operation on fractures of the radius and ulna and found that there were seventeen instances of non-union out of seventy-eight fractures operated within the first six days, and no cases of non-union in fifty-two fractures operated after the first seven days. In a larger series of fractures of the forearm bones the experience of Smith and Sage (1957), on the other hand, does not confirm this observation.

Adly Guindy,[1] working in my clinic, has repeated this investigation of the time elapsing between fracture and internal fixation, in relation to successful osseous union, in the case of thirty-eight fractures of the shaft of the femur treated by intramedullary nailing. His findings, though admittedly on a very small number of cases, support the idea that delayed interference is beneficial; six patients required bone-grafting out of twenty-four operated within the first week of the injury (25 per cent.) whereas only one patient out of fourteen operated more than one week after the injury required a bone-graft (7 per cent.). In the cases operated by internal fixation more than one week after the injury the amount of callus in the radiograph at three months was greater than in those operated within the first week after injury.

While absolute proof is still lacking that it is better to delay operation than to intervene urgently, at least it has been shown that no harm is done by delayed intervention. This observation would seem to be consistent with ideas on the blood supply of the fractured cortical bones, because it suggests that to delay intervention might give time for reactive hyperæmia to start in the ends of the bones. If operative intervention is performed urgently it may obstruct the action of blood to already partially ischæmic bone ends and delay their invasion by the hyperæmic process which precedes healing.

If delayed intervention is postponed too long (*i.e.*, more than two or three weeks) this will increase the technical difficulties of the operation by obscuring the detail of the bone ends and making it impossible to match them for a hair-line fit. In transverse fractures of the shaft of the femur which defy manipulative reduction due to gross swelling of the thigh, a delay long enough to absorb effused blood and lose some muscle bulk greatly facilitates the operation. This type of fracture frequently occurs in athletic young men whose bulky thigh muscles offer a serious obstacle to exposure of the fragment. In these cases I now rarely operate before the expiry of two weeks. Easy operations have fewer complications than difficult operations.

REFERENCES

CHARNLEY, J. (1953). *Compression Arthrodesis.* Edinburgh: E. & S. Livingstone.
CHARNLEY, J. & BAKER, S. L. (1952). *J. Bone Jt Surg.* **34B**, 187.
EGGERS, G. W., STEINDLER, T. O. & POINEVAT, C. M. (1949). *J. Bone Jt Surg.* **31A**, 693.
FRIEDENBERG, Z. B. & FRENCH, G. (1952). *Surg. Gynec. Obstet.* **94**, 743.
PHEMISTER, D. B. (1947). *J. Bone Jt Surg.* **29**, 946.
SMITH, HUGH & SAGE, FRED. P. (1957). *J. Bone Jt Surg.* **39A**, 91.
SMITH, J. E. M. (1959). *J. Bone Jt Surg.* **41B**, 122.
URIST, M. R. & JOHNSON, W. (1943). *J. Bone Jt Surg.* **25**, 375.
URIST, M. R., MAZET, ROBERT, Jun. & McLEAN, F. C. (1954). *J. Bone Jt Surg.* **36A**, 931.

[1] In press.

CHAPTER TWO

THE MECHANICS OF CONSERVATIVE
TREATMENT

DESCRIPTIONS of operative technique are to be found in most modern textbooks of fracture treatment, and often in great detail; by comparison the details of manipulative technique are usually indicated in only the vaguest of general outlines. This is not surprising if manipulative treatment is regarded as an art rather than as a science, because an art is essentially something which defies description and is therefore to be learned only by practice and apprenticeship.

In this chapter an attempt is made to reveal the scientific basis of manipulative methods. Unless the teacher of manipulative technique is able to create a *mental picture* of a manipulation, the student may waste months of experience and much valuable material before he eventually discovers what others may long have known but have failed to communicate. These mental pictures should not be decried by an experienced operator if the interpretations here offered seem to him open to question; the student must adapt these pictures to suit impressions gained from his own practical experience and they will thus form a useful basis on which to build.

The Soft Tissues associated with a Fracture

When the student inspects the radiograph of a badly displaced fracture, such as that of a Pott's fracture of the ankle, he may well despair at the thought of manipulative reduction. Manual reduction of a case such as that illustrated in Fig. 38 would appear not unlike the assembling of a jig-saw puzzle in the dark. The solution of the difficulty emerges, and the precision of reduction is realised, only when the supreme importance of the soft tissues is appreciated. The importance of the soft tissues is often forgotten because these are not seen in an X-ray. Bone fragments are to be regarded as of secondary importance to the damaged and undamaged soft parts; *the mere fracture of a bone does not determine the displacement of its fragments*. When displacement is present certain soft parts have been ruptured and conversely certain other soft parts usually remain intact; it is the latter which give the clue to the reduction. If the undamaged soft parts are brought into normal relationship, the bone fragments will return to their normal positions. The action of soft tissues in guiding displaced fragments back to their normal position is demonstrated in the fractured femur illustrated in Fig. 39.

43

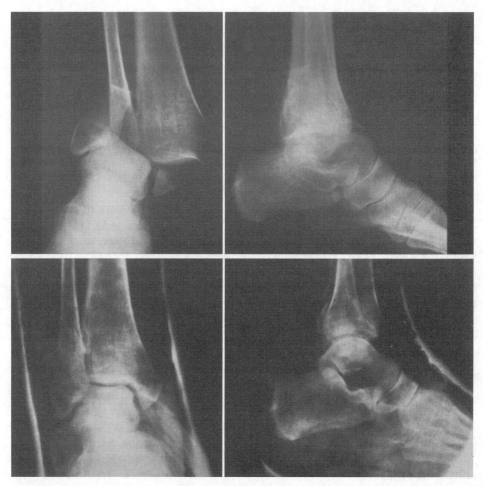

FIG. 38

Anatomical reduction by closed manipulation. Without knowledge of the role of the intact soft tissues, the reduction of this injury might appear a forlorn hope.

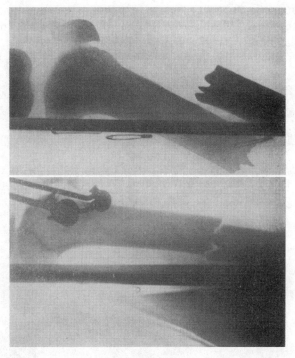

FIG. 39

Reduction of overriding fracture of the femur produced by
a single movement of traction under general anæsthesia.
This alignment is produced through the mediation of the
intact soft parts.

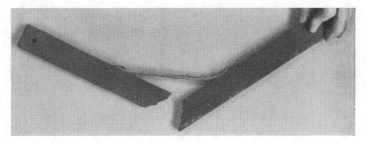

FIG. 40

Model, consisting of two pieces of wood connected by a strip of leather,
represents the fragments of a fractured long bone which are connected
on the concave side of the deformity by intact periosteum and fibrous
structures. If the existence of this soft-tissue hinge is forgotten, because
it is radio-translucent, the apposing of the fragments by blind manipulation would be a matter of pure chance.

45

In the model illustrated in Fig. 40 it might be thought impossible to expect an anatomical reduction of this 'fracture' without some assistance from the eye; but by using the intact fibrous elements on the concave side of the 'fracture' (indicated in the model by the strip of leather) it is possible, even blindfold, to guide the fragments into their anatomical position (Fig. 41). This model

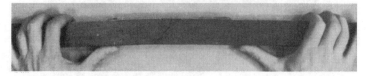

FIG. 41

Showing how the soft-tissue hinge, on the concave side of the deformity, can guide the fragments into position. The applied forces are tending to over-correct the deformity; this puts the tissue hinge under tension and compresses the bone ends against each other. The three-point system.

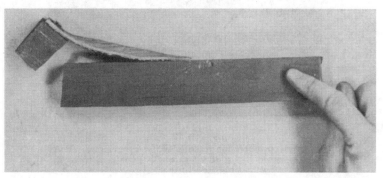

A

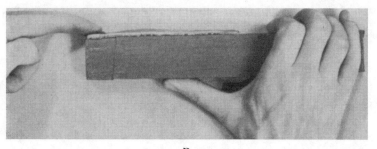

B
FIG. 42

Model illustrating the soft-tissue hinge in fractures at the extremities of long bones, *e.g.*, Colles', Pott's, and supracondylar fractures of the humerus.

represents **the mechanism of the soft tissue 'hinge' common to the majority of fractures.** A similar model illustrating the reduction of fractures such as the Colles', Pott's, and supracondylar fractures of humerus, is illustrated

46

in Fig. 42, A and B. These models show why it is almost impossible to over-reduce these fractures; because *the intact fibrous tissues on the concave side of the original deformity prevent over-reduction unless the force used is so great that it ruptures them* (Fig. 43).

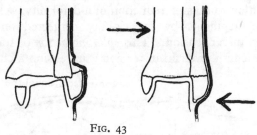

FIG. 43

Showing how it is usually impossible to over-reduce fractures such as the Colles' or the Pott's. The tension in the intact structures on the concave side prevents over-correction. Faulty reduction of the Pott's fracture may sometimes be traced to a fear of over-displacement.

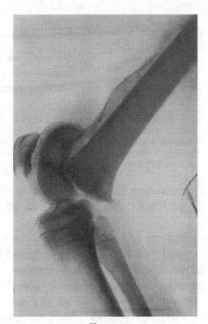

FIG. 44

Five-weeks-old displacement of the lower femoral epiphysis; ossification in the periosteum visibly demonstrating the soft-tissue hinge. The soft tissues are to be regarded as a tube from which the shaft of the femur has escaped into the popliteal space through a posterior tear. (*Mr Palin's case.*)

Visual evidence of the existence of the soft-tissue 'hinge' is demonstrated in the slipped lower femoral epiphysis in Fig. 44 where the periosteum on the concave side of the deformity has become ossified in the relaxed position.

Traction

The value of traction has long been known in the reduction of many fractures. Traction produces a reduction through the surrounding soft parts which align the fragments by their tension. Continuous traction, generated by weights and pulleys, in addition to causing reduction of a deformity, will also produce a *relative fixation* of the fragments by the rigidity conferred on the surrounding soft structures when under tension. This *splinting action* of traction can be illustrated by observing a length of chain in tension; in tension a chain behaves like a solid

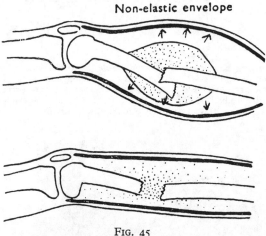

Non-elastic envelope

FIG. 45

Illustrating hydraulic obstruction to traction when a iimb is grossly swollen. If the inelastic fibrous capsule tends to assume a spherical shape the length of the limb must decrease. When the effusion absorbs and the muscles waste, over-distraction occurs.

bar, the individual links possessing no relative motion, but without tension the movement of one link is no longer communicated to its neighbour and so each link is relatively mobile.

Were it not for the stretching of soft parts (with consequent separation of the bone ends), it could be argued that the use of continuous traction would instantly solve **the fundamental problem of closed fracture treatment: how to secure fixation of the fracture and yet preserve joint function.** By continuous traction, alignment can be maintained while at the same time it is possible to devise apparatus permitting joint movement. In those cases where over-distraction cannot precipitate delayed union, *i.e.*, the long oblique fractures where slight over-pulling does not abolish bone contact, methods using continuous traction are rational and acceptable.

In reviewing the action of traction we must consider the nature of the elements which offer resistance to elongation. The most obvious resistance to traction is that of muscular tone; but the difficulty which is so often encountered in securing full length under anæsthesia shows at once that muscular tone cannot be the most important factor.

In some cases a *hydraulic element* is present which resists elongation. Closed fractures, in which there has been a large effusion of blood, demonstrate this hydraulic mechanism; for in these the fibrous compartments of the limb, becoming distended and turgid, offer a rigid barrier to elongation. This mechanism is best seen in fractures of the shaft of the femur where, following hæmorrhage into the muscles, the thigh tries to adopt a spherical shape (because a sphere has the greatest capacity for a fixed surface area) and therefore in order to become greater in width the thigh must become shorter in length (Fig. 45). In such cases the effusion is sometimes so great that it is difficult to slide the ring of a Thomas splint over the swollen thigh. By allowing a period of a week or ten days to

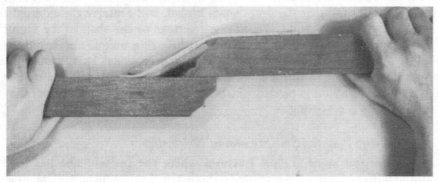

FIG. 46

Showing obstruction to traction by the soft-tissue hinge when the fragments are interlocked. Strong traction will rupture the periosteal bridge with possible serious consequences to union. By increasing the initial deformity this interlocking can be released without using traction.

elapse before a second attempt at remanipulation it may be possible to secure a reduction when the thigh has become soft by the fluid being partly resorbed; open reduction, however, would be the ideal procedure.

Another mechanism offering a rigid barrier to elongation results from the *interlocking of soft tissues*. This mechanism was demonstrated by Beveridge Moore (1928) in experimental fractures of fresh, periosteum-covered, animal bones. The model in Fig. 46 illustrates this mechanism; reduction of this artificial fracture can be obtained only by increasing the original deformity in order to release the bone ends. Violent axis traction could reduce this fracture only by rupturing the last remaining strands of periosteum connecting the bone ends, a factor which has often been suggested as a reason for non-union.

Classification of Fracture by the Mechanics of Fixation

It is instructive to classify fractures according to the physical conditions best suited to their fixation. Three groups can be distinguished by their **varying degrees of stability to a telescoping force applied after reduction:**

1. *Fractures without Stability against Shortening*

These comprise the oblique or spiral and the comminuted fractures. In these some form of traction would be necessary if it were desired to prevent the shortening which results from the unopposed action of muscular tone (unless the fracture is strutted by another bone lying at its side).

2. *Fractures with Complete Stability against Shortening*

These are the transverse fractures. Once the bone ends of a transverse fracture are manipulated into some degree of end-to-end contact, the fracture immediately becomes stable against shortening. **Transverse fractures need splintage only to control angular deformity.** If plaster of Paris be used, the cast will act merely as a mould to ensure that the limb, when healed, will preserve the external shape imposed on it by the splint. Transverse fractures of the shaft of the femur are, however, unsuited to this form of treatment through a unique circumstance : the shrinkage of the thigh muscles, which possess exceptional bulk, would allow a fracture of the femur to slip if it were treated from the outset in plaster ; in the fractured femur a splint is needed which can retain continuous control of the thigh while shrinkage is occurring.

3. *Fractures with Potential Stability against Shortening*

These are the blunt oblique fractures where the fracture line lies less than 45 degrees from the transverse line. These are the commonest of all fractures and therefore some knowledge of theoretical mechanics is valuable, even though this theory may not be capable of practical application on every occasion.

It is in this group that stability against shortening can be obtained by using knowledge gained from an understanding of the soft-tissue ' hinge.'

If a blunt oblique fracture is reduced by manipulation and is then slightly *angulated in the direction of over-correction*, the intact soft-tissue hinge will be put into slight tension. Under these conditions the bone ends will be pressed together *and the fracture will retain some stability to a telescoping force while the hinge is in tension.* This action of the soft-tissue hinge, assisted by an almost intact fibula, is well illustrated in the fractured tibia in Fig. 47. Tension in the soft-tissue hinge can be maintained by applying a plaster moulded to *over-correct* the original angulation. This is illustrated in Fig. 48, A and B, which also demonstrates **the paradox that a ' curved ' plaster is necessary in order to make a straight limb.** In this type of fracture it is erroneous to regard a plaster merely as a passive mould exerting an even pressure over the whole surface of the contained limb. **The ' three-point ' plaster exerts pressure at certain precisely determined points on the skeleton and none at others.** Typical examples of plasters demonstrating three-point systems are illustrated in Fig. 49 for the Pott's, Colles', and Bennett's fractures where the pressure points are indicated which constitute three-point systems.

In localising the points of a three-point system it will be seen that *two of the three points are those where the surgeon's hands moulded the plaster while setting ;*

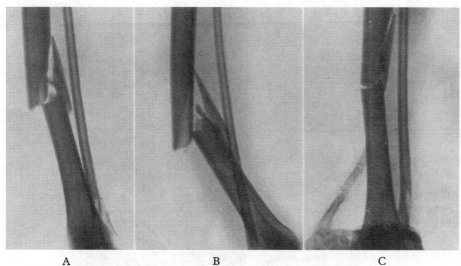

A   B   C

Fig. 47

A, Fracture of the tibia and fibula before reduction.
B, Appearance on applying a valgus force to distal fragments.
C, Appearance on applying a varus force to distal fragments.
The ruptured tissues are therefore situated on the medial aspect and the intact tissue hinge is on the lateral aspect. (*Essex-Lopresti, Birmingham Accident Hospital.*)

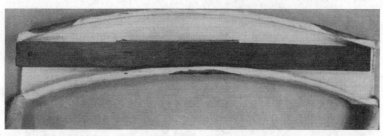

A

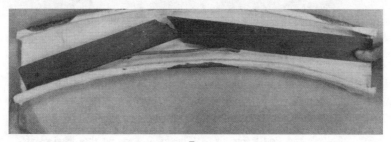

B

Fig. 48

A, Showing how a three-point splint can hold a reduction by keeping the soft-tissue hinge under tension. This model consists of a curved plaster gutter, to represent the plaster cast, and thus illustrates the paradox that on principle it is necessary to have a curved plaster in order to secure a straight limb.
B, Showing how a fracture will redisplace if the three-point splint is applied in the wrong direction, *i.e.*, allowing the soft-tissue hinge to become slack.

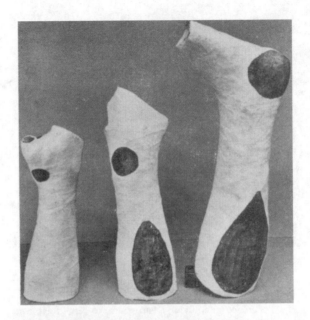

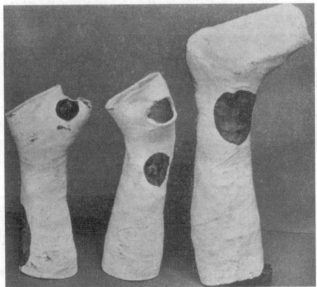

Fig. 49

Examples of three-point action in common plasters—Bennett's, Colles', and Pott's fractures. The small areas on the distal parts of the casts represent the forces applied by the surgeon's hands to the proximal and distal fragments. The large areas on the proximal parts of the casts represent the third point which renders the reduction stable when the surgeon's hands are removed.

one is applied to the proximal fragment while the other is applied to the distal fragment. But though the action of the surgeon's hands maintains a reduction by *two* forces, it is impossible to hold a reduction by *two* forces alone if these are applied by an inanimate object such as a splint. If a splint is applied which exerts pressure at only two points, the reduction will slip because the splint can move

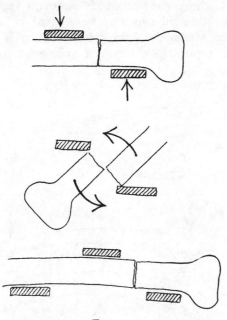

FIG. 50

Showing how a two-point system (*i.e.*, forces applied only to the proximal and distal fragments) is unstable. If the fracture rotates in the direction of the 'couple' produced by these two forces, then redisplacement will occur. By introducing a third force to neutralise this couple the system becomes stable.

away from the fracture (rotating in the opposite direction to the 'couple' produced by these two forces) (Fig. 50). It is necessary, therefore, to introduce a third force in order to neutralise this turning couple and so to prevent the plaster from rotating away from the limb. In the plasters illustrated in Fig. 49 it will be seen that *the third point extends over a diffuse area at the proximal part of the cast.*

Padded and Unpadded Plasters

An understanding of the three-point action of a plaster splint elucidates the similarity of padded and unpadded plasters. There has been a tendency in some quarters to regard the unpadded, or 'skin-tight,' plaster as the only logical form of fixation, and to regard padded plasters as outmoded and ineffective. In actual fact the only *mechanical* difference between padded and unpadded plasters is one of degree, and concerns the amount of 'molecular' movement possible at the fracture line. The skin-tight plaster provides better immobilisation of the fracture, as judged by the amount of movement which is possible between the cells of the healing callus. But even in a skin-tight plaster the amount of immobilisation is only relative, owing to the movement which can occur between the skin and the skeleton. True immobilisation can only be secured by some form of internal fixation. Even in the accurately fitting plaster which is usually applied for a fracture of the carpal scaphoid, a patient can wriggle his wrist by at least ⅛ inch in relation to the cast.

As regards the prevention of massive movement at a fracture line (*i.e.*, complete

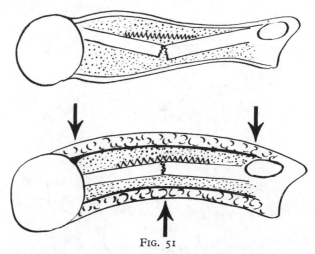

FIG. 51

Showing that a skin-tight plaster, beautifully moulded to the external shape of a limb, is capable of allowing redisplacement to occur because it does not exert a three-point action. On the other hand, a padded plaster is capable of preventing redisplacement, provided that it is moulded into the correct three-point forces.

redisplacement of the fracture), there is no essential difference between padded and unpadded plasters, *provided that they both exhibit three-point action.* If a fracture of the radius and ulna were to slip in a padded plaster, it is erroneous to think that this accident might have been prevented had the cast been unpadded. **If a fracture slips in a well applied padded plaster, then that fracture was mechanically unsuitable for treatment by plaster and another mechanical principle should have been chosen.**

Perhaps the most common example of failure to understand the three-point action of plaster is seen in the treatment of greenstick fractures of the forearm by skin-tight plasters. A greenstick fracture illustrates more clearly than any other the action of a strong fibrous tissue 'hinge' on the concave side of the 'lead-pipe' deformity (Fig. 51). It is obvious that three forces must be applied to manipulate such a deformed forearm into correct alignment; but it is often not appreciated that **alignment cannot be safely controlled by a plaster slab applied only to one aspect of the forearm.** It is quite true that hundreds of such cases throughout the country are every week successfully treated by this procedure even though mechanically it is essentially unsound; but in many other cases serious recurrence of the original deformity will occur. **A single plaster slab is incapable of three-point action.**

But even if a complete plaster is applied to a greenstick fracture of the forearm, *the lead-pipe deformity can still recur inside the plaster unless the cast is moulded to have a slight curvature in the direction of over-correction of the original deformity.* This recurrence of angulation inside an unpadded plaster can be imagined as being caused by the tissue hinge behaving as though it were a piece of stretched elastic; the tension of the hinge forces the bones towards their original deformity, and the soft muscles interposed between the bones and the cast offer no resistance to this displacement, even though the plaster is skin-tight. This movement in the direction of the original displacement shows that **a padded plaster positively moulded into a three-point action is mechanically superior to an unpadded cast with a neutral or simple ' encasing ' function.**

It is instructive to compare the two plaster casts illustrated in Fig. 52 in which one is a good copy of the external shape of the ankle and the other looks to be a very clumsy and inexpert product. As will be explained in the treatment of the Pott's fracture, the ugly cast is in reality the better cast, because it bears the impress of the surgeon's hands moulding the displaced fragments into position.

The tendency to recurrence of the original deformity in a greenstick fracture of the forearm can be prevented by deliberately completing the greenstick fracture, thereby rupturing the intact soft parts which in a child act like a spring to reassert the original deformity. I am often asked whether or not one should make a green-stick fracture of the forearm complete as a routine procedure. The answer is that one must always *over-correct* any fracture during reduction; if a greenstick fracture of the forearm cannot be overcorrected without completing the fracture, then the fracture must be completed. If the deformity can be over-corrected without the fracture being complete, it need not be completed if the surgeon understands how to model the plaster to keep a three point system acting on the reduced fracture.

Late Deformity

In fracture treatment *late deformities* are a constant hazard; they cause anxiety for both surgeon and patient alike. Here, to be forewarned is to be forearmed. If a surgeon maintains a conscious anticipation of late deformity throughout the post-reduction phases of treatment he will almost always be able to prevent it; it is when the surgeon is unaware of the latent dangers of the method he is using that late deformity takes him by surprise. To anticipate late deformity it is necessary to know the *common patterns* of deformity as they present themselves in particular instances, as well as to have an understanding of the mechanism of late deformity in general.

Late deformity is rendered more than ordinarily probable whenever delayed

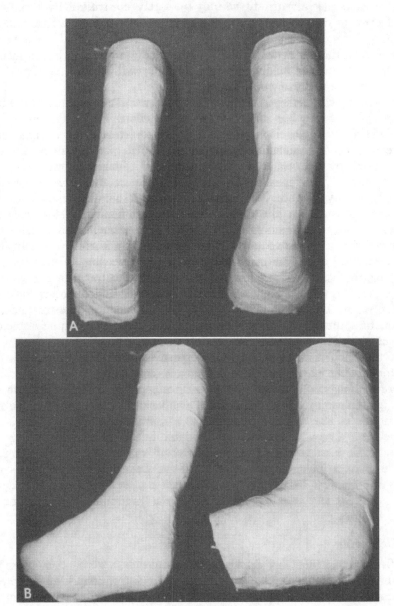

FIG. 52

The plaster on the left, used for a Pott's fracture, is more elegant than that
on the right; it is however much less effective because that on the right is
moulded to produce a 'three-point' system of forces. The indentations
caused by the moulding force of the surgeon's hands can be seen above and
below the ankle.

consolidation complicates the healing of a fracture. If a fracture consolidates rapidly, a good result is practically certain even in an apparatus of second-rate mechanical design. If delayed consolidation supervenes, the same apparatus may permit late angulation, because the patient becomes restless and active just at the stage when the apparatus is beginning to reveal its mechanical faults. The maintenance of correct alignment in the presence of delayed union is a very stringent test of sound design in any system of splintage. If delayed union were to be more common even than it is, unsuspected mechanical defects would be revealed in many of the routine methods which give good results in everyday practice. In the weight-bearing extremities *late angulation due to the action of superincumbent body weight is so obvious that it will be omitted from this analysis.* The late deformity to be considered here is the 'spontaneous' late deformity which develops while the patient is still in bed or still in a plaster.

There are two main factors to be considered in spontaneous late deformity: (1) the force of gravity and (2) the force of muscular tone. Gravity can act in various ways according to the method used for treatment; the action of muscular tone results from the *superior pull of one muscle group over another*. Both these forces can generate enhanced power to bend the callus through the action of leverage systems, which can roughly be calculated from measurements of the length of the bony fragments, as will be demonstrated in subsequent paragraphs.

In addition to these causes of late angulation, experience shows that certain types of apparatus have a tendency to modify the late deformity according to certain constantly recurring patterns. It is unnecessary to anticipate late angulation towards any of the four directions of the compass but merely to anticipate it in those directions for which the fracture and the method of treatment are notorious. A few examples of common late deformity patterns can be enumerated:

Pertrochanteric fractures of femur (any splint) .	late varus.
Midshaft femur (on Thomas splint) . . .	late varus.
Lower quarter shaft of femur (Thomas splint) .	often a late valgus.
Radius and ulna (in plaster)	late ulnar convexity, radial concavity.
Humerus (in hanging cast)	late varus.
Colles' fracture (dorsal slab)	late valgus.

Example 1

It is a clinical fact that transverse fractures of the shaft of the femur are prone to late angulation far more frequently than long oblique fractures. This can be explained by comparing the relative forces exerted on the callus in these two types of fracture as the following analysis will show.

In Fig. 53 is depicted an oblique fracture of the femur A and a transverse fracture B, which are both held rigidly by their proximal ends while an angulating force X is applied to the femoral condyles.

In case A the oblique fracture occupies a length of the shaft equal to six times its diameter. The upper limit of the fracture is situated twelve times the diameter of the shaft from its lower end. C represents the levers involved, if it be assumed that the fulcrum is sited at the proximal part of the fracture. The leverage acting under these assumptions is, therefore, in the proportion of 12 to 6, and thus the force on the callus at the distal part of the fracture is 2X.

In the case of the femur B, the transverse fracture is situated at twelve times the diameter of the shaft from the lower end. D represents the levers involved, if it be assumed that the fulcrum is situated at the cortex under compression. Thus a leverage in the proportion of 12 to 1 is available to separate the callus at the part of the cortex which is under tension. The angulating force is thus six times greater in the transverse case than in the oblique case.

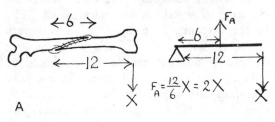

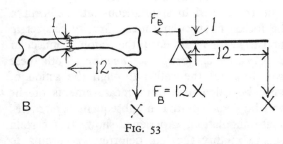

This enhanced leverage in the transverse case acts, moreover, on a fracture which has only a sixth of the area of the oblique case; *thus each unit area of callus in the transverse fracture is subjected to thirty-six times the strain in the oblique fracture* in the hypothetical case under consideration.

FIG. 53

Applying the same type of mechanical analysis, it is instructive to contrast the magnitude of the forces causing late angulation in a fracture of the shaft of a femur with those causing angulation in a fracture of the proximal phalanx of a finger.

Example 2

Consider the case of a transverse fracture at the junction of the middle and upper thirds of the shaft of the femur (Fig. 54). If a guillotine amputation were to be performed through the line of the fracture, the detached limb might weigh some 20 lb. The centre of gravity of this mass would lie about 2 inches below the knee joint which, in turn, would lie about 14 inches below the fracture line in a person of average height. If the diameter of the shaft of the femur be taken

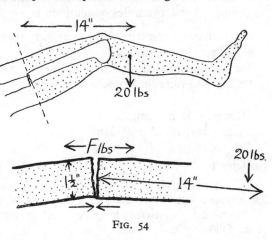

FIG. 54

as $1\frac{1}{4}$ inches, and if it be considered that the shaft angulates by pivoting at the cortex under compression (the concave side), then a linear force will be present at the cortex under tension (the convex side) of:

$$\frac{14}{1\cdot25} \times 20 = 220 \text{ lb.}$$

It is not difficult to understand, therefore, why plates bend, screws pull out, and grafts break, if the fracture is not united by the time the force of gravity, uncounter-balanced, takes hold of the weight of the limb distal to the fracture.

This explanation shows how a badly designed plaster, by increasing the weight of the distal fragment and failing to take a secure hold of the proximal fragment, can in some cases actually increase a natural tendency to late angulation. If a plaster support were to be needed for a fracture of the lower third of the femur, it is then obvious that a 'long leg' plaster would be worse than useless because its weight would invite late angulation.

Example 3

Consider now the forces acting on a transverse fracture of the proximal phalanx of a *finger* calculated in the same way as the preceding. The distal fragment is to be taken as 1 inch in length and the diameter of the bone as $\frac{1}{4}$ inch. The weight of the digit, estimated as if it were amputated by guillotine through the fracture line, can be taken as $\frac{1}{16}$ lb. Gravity will thus exert an angulating force on the unsplinted fracture which tends to separate the cortices on the convex side with a force of:

$$\frac{1}{\cdot 25} \times \frac{1}{16} = \frac{1}{4} \text{ lb.}$$

It can thus be argued that callus in a fracture of a finger is subjected to forces (*as a result of gravity alone*) of only one eight-hundredth part of the forces acting on a fracture of the shaft of the femur *even before weight-bearing is allowed*.

Example 4

Some idea of why nature depends for union of the shafts of long bones on the production of periosteal callus can be gleaned from the following mechanical study.

Consider again the figures calculated for the transverse fracture of the femoral shaft in Example 2. With the shaft of the femur measuring $1\frac{1}{4}$ inches in diameter and the total weight of the limb distal to the fracture weighing 20 lb., it was shown that a tearing force of 220 lb. is exerted on the callus on the convex side of the deformity. But if nature encloses the fracture site in a bulky mass of periosteal callus which measures a total diameter of 3 inches, it will become evident that the strain on the most peripheral part of the ensheathing callus is much reduced and becomes only:

$$\frac{14}{3} \times 20 = 90 \text{ lb.}$$

This principle of placing a weak structure at a considerable distance from the centre of angulation is well known to constructional engineers and underlies the principle of the 'stressed skin' construction of aircraft, by which a thin sheet of metal placed on the outside of an aircraft wing becomes as strong as a heavy girder of steel used as a central spar. From such considerations one feels that endosteal callus cannot be an important element in the early healing of fractures of the shafts of the long bones.

CHAPTER THREE

JOINT MOVEMENT IN CONSERVATIVE
METHODS

PERFECT anatomical restoration and perfect freedom of joint movement can be obtained simultaneously only by internal fixation. It is possible to argue that most of the difficulties of closed fracture treatment can be traced to the prevention of joint stiffness. Closed methods can offer anatomical restoration only if the start of joint movement is delayed. It is the significance of delay in starting joint movement which is the crucial point in understanding closed methods.

The ultimate recovery of full joint function after a fracture depends on many factors and not only on early exercise. This is suggested by the fact that the end results of conservative treatment, after a slow start, can often be surprisingly good, while those of operative methods, after a very promising start, can sometimes be disappointing. It is therefore obvious that we must review the factors which govern the recovery of joint movement following a fracture, so far as we know them.

In studying the stiffness of a joint following a fracture of an associated bone the greatest danger to the furtherance of knowledge is the too facile acceptance of simple mechanistic explanations. It is probable that the processes concerned with the recovery of joint function are of great biological complexity. Too often there is a tendency to think of stiff joints in terms of stiff engine-bearings or of rusty door-hinges and, with this childlike concept, to devise apparatus to loosen the stiffness by repeated mechanical movements. This mechanistic interpretation of organic processes is inherent in many popular physiotherapeutic measures; the use of kneading massage 'to break up fibrositic nodules,' the softening of areas of induration by heat, the dispersal of œdema by stroking, the restoration of flexibility by inuncting oil, etc., are but few of the simple ways in which the tissues are imagined as lumps in pastry, or as wax to be softened by warmth, as wood to be made pliable with water, or as leather to be made flexible with oil.

In reviewing the facts concerning joint rehabilitation, it is surprising what little direct experimental evidence we have at our disposal and how scanty is our knowledge of the normal physiology of joint function. In the subsequent paragraphs evidence will be produced to support the writer's opinion that in closed treatment the prevention of joint stiffness by early joint movement may not be based on such sound biological fact as might at first sight be imagined.

It is hoped to show that **the late exercise of joints is part of the natural fracture healing process, and is compatible with normal healing processes.**

The Fixation of Joints in Plaster

We are now able to review in true perspective the massed experience of a decade (1930-40) during which the skin-tight plaster was extensively used in Britain according to the doctrine expounded by Böhler. In this teaching the joints above and below the fracture were immobilised in skin-tight plaster for just so long as it took the fracture to unite. If delayed union developed this fixation was continued over many months. It was Böhler's contention that no permanent joint stiffness would result from prolonged plaster fixation, provided that the joints were in the optimum position for function, and provided that the limb was actively employed in the performance of useful work while in its cast. This theory maintained that the static contraction of muscles would maintain the intercellular circulation and so prevent the stagnation and œdema which was regarded as favouring fibroplasia, which was regarded as the explanation of permanent loss of flexibility in joint capsules. Böhler went even so far as to declare that plaster fixation was imperative as an insurance against stiffness, and he believed that surgeons not understanding this were risking avoidable and permanent disability in their patients. *It is interesting and instructive to observe that this teaching put no emphasis on physiotherapy or special rehabilitation after removal of plaster*; it was believed that a patient should be able to walk out of his plaster with little or no disability if reablement while in plaster had been effectively carried out. To this end the patient was taught to perform exercises involving considerable physical exertion while still in plaster (*i.e.*, fractured spines in casts were taught to carry weights of 40 kg.). These enthusiastic claims for the conservative treatment of fractures by plaster are perhaps somewhat overdrawn, but in discarding those parts of his theories which in the light of further experience we now know to be false, we must not make the mistake of overlooking the great content of fundamental truth. The teaching of Böhler in part has failed, but it has not failed on the score of producing joint stiffness; **the teaching of Böhler failed only because it did not eliminate delayed union.** In challenging theories of plaster fixation we must remember that **the majority of joints treated in plaster do eventually recover their full range of movement** though there may often be some delay.

In considering the problems of joint stiffness resulting from plaster fixation we must isolate from discussion those cases in which sepsis or nerve injury has been present. **The commonest single cause of permanent joint stiffness is sepsis;** the stiffness caused by the dense scar tissue left by sepsis is irreparable.

It is probable also that we must use with caution the specific example of the stiff knee joint following a fractured femur; the study of stiffness in this joint after a fracture of the femur sheds much light on joint function, but the stiffness of this joint occurs more readily and is more resistant to treatment than is the stiffness of almost any other joint: its example must therefore not be allowed to influence unduly the whole subject of plaster fixation. This tendency in surgical science, to allow a rather special example to be applied as a general principle, is one against which we must be continually on our guard (a similar instance of faulty deduction is in the example of the fractured carpal scaphoid which is allowed to influence adversely the treatment of many trivial fractures). In contrast to the knee joint, the speed with which the wrist joint almost invariably recovers its full range after many months of plaster fixation is always a most striking observation and, while taking longer to recover, the radius and ulna, and the tibia and fibula, also *eventually* recover practically full range in their associated joints after more than six months of continuous plaster fixation.

The experimental fixation of joints in plaster has been investigated by numerous workers and the literature is reviewed by Scaglietti and Casuccio (1935). These workers found that in dogs no serious and irreparable joint changes could be demonstrated after several months of continuous plaster fixation. Those parts of the articular surfaces which were in contact with each other always remained healthy, but those parts of the articular surfaces which were in contact with the joint capsule developed superficial ulcers. It appears that **the persistence of normal joint histology is probably the result of continuous minute movement which can never be abolished by plaster fixation.**

While it is probable that the fixation of joints in plaster does neither serious harm nor material good, there can be no doubt of its value in the treatment of fresh compound fractures. The recovery of function after prolonged plaster fixation in this type of injury is to be observed in the work of Trueta. The excellent joint function after the closed plaster treatment of compound injuries is the result of eliminating or minimising sepsis and so *eliminating one of the most sinister causes of permanent stiffness.* Our modern interest in chemotherapy must never allow us to forget that rest is and always will be a fundamental surgical principle.

STIFFNESS OF THE KNEE FOLLOWING FRACTURES OF THE FEMORAL SHAFT

The stiffness of the knee which is such a notorious complication of fractures of the femoral shaft is an exceptionally interesting subject for study. After a fracture of the shaft of the femur the knee stiffens more readily, and takes longer to recover its full movement, than probably any other joint in the body (with the exception, possibly, of the elbow); but even so it should not be imagined that the stiff knee after a fracture of the femoral shaft, troublesome though it is, has always a hopeless prognosis. It is a surprising thing about the knee joint that continuous recovery of movement often proceeds for as long as eighteen months after the start of full weight-bearing. This late recovery is quite unlike the behaviour of most other stiff joints which rarely increase by a significant range after the first six months of rehabilitation. The function of weight-bearing seems vital to the late recovery of knee range; but here, again, those cases where stiffness is due to sepsis after compound fractures of the femur must be eliminated from the discussion, because in these the stiffness is caused by scar tissue too dense to absorb, and knee stiffness in these cases rarely improves after six months.

Intra-articular versus Extra-articular Causes of Knee Stiffness after a Fractured Femoral Shaft

Six lines of evidence can be adduced in favour of the theory that the limitation of knee movement which follows a fracture of the femur is mainly the result of extra-articular adhesions ; these are :

1. COMPARISON WITH FRACTURES OF THE TIBIA AND FIBULA

Owing to the common occurrence of delayed union in fracture of the tibia treated by conservative methods it frequently happens that the knee has to be fixed in

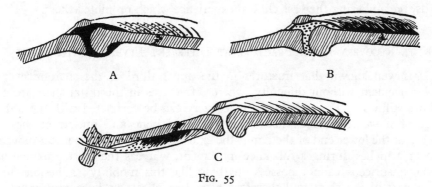

FIG. 55

A, Illustrates orthodox concept of knee stiffness after fracture of shaft of the femur as due to articular adhesions.

B, Indicates author's concept of stiffness due to 'master' adhesions in the quadriceps with only soft 'secondary' adhesions in the joint.

C, Illustrates tendency of the ankle to stiffen after fracture of the tibia, *but not of the knee*, even after prolonged fixation in plaster, when the fracture does not involve the quadriceps.

plaster for six months or more ; yet little or no difficulty is experienced in achieving 90 degrees of motion in a few weeks and often full knee range is secured by that time. The different behaviour of the knee joint after this duration of fixation in fractures of the femur is quite remarkable and would seem to indicate that the involvement of the quadriceps muscle in scar tissue might be the deciding factor (Fig. 55, A, B, C). In fractures of the tibia it is not uncommon to find stiffness of the ankle joint persisting for many weeks whereas this is not a common complication of fractures of the femoral shaft.

2. INJURIES OF THE KNEE JOINT UNACCOMPANIED BY FRACTURE OF THE FEMUR

When severe injuries to the ligaments of the knee are treated by immobilisation in plaster for three or four months the rapidity and completeness of recovery of knee function are often astonishing. Sir Robert Jones has commented on the good knee function which is usually obtained after complete dislocation of the knee in the following terms :

' The interesting fact is that, in spite of the extensive rupture of ligaments, including the crucial ligaments, the functional results in recorded cases have been so good. The explanation of this is that the lesion is so formidable that prolonged fixation is absolutely necessary; early use and movement is impossible without displacement occurring. Hence torn structures are usually given time to unite firmly, and with exercise and use considerable freedom of movement is recovered in time. . . . The great lesson seems to be that if the displacement is reduced and the limb fixed in a straight position, nature will do surprisingly well.'

Those who tend to decry conservative methods would do well to mark these words, remembering the vast clinical experience which promoted them.

3. KNEE RECOVERY AFTER FRACTURE AT DIFFERENT LEVELS OF THE SHAFT

It is well known that fractures in the upper third of the shaft recover full knee movement without difficulty, whereas fractures in the distal shaft are prone to knee stiffness. This difference in recovery can be correlated with the different range of movement which takes place between bone and muscle at these two levels ; at the lower end of the femur the extensor apparatus has a linear movement of 2 or 3 inches during a full knee movement, whereas the most proximal fibres of the quadriceps cannot possess anything like this mobility ; adhesions in the upper part of the shaft will therefore have less effect on knee movement than they will at the lower level.

Against this explanation the fact is sometimes advanced that troublesome knee stiffness is encountered after arthrodesis of the hip where the quadriceps muscle is not involved. It must not be forgotten, however, that knee stiffness in these cases is only permanent in the elderly patient and this results, presumably, from the fixation of an abnormal joint.

4. FRACTURES OF THE PATELLA DURING MANIPULATION

Manipulation to secure more flexion in the knee after a fracture of the femoral shaft is often complicated by fracture of the decalcified patella. This fact would seem to indicate that the main resistance to flexion lies proximal to the patella, because flexion of the knee is secured with very little further effort after the patella has fractured. The intra-articular adhesions would, therefore, appear to be soft, whereas the adhesions in the extensor apparatus are dense. It is therefore reasonable to suggest that adhesions in the quadriceps are the ' master ' adhesions and that intra-articular adhesions are secondary to the enforced fixation of the knee (Fig. 56).

5. RESULTS OF PLASTIC OPERATIONS ON THE QUADRICEPS

Good results have been reported following excision of the adherent vastus intermedius at the level of the fracture as described by T. C. Thompson (1944). The operation offers a good chance of securing 90 degrees in knees which previously were very stiff. The procedure is often combined with incisions into the capsule of the knee joint in order to divide the lateral and medial expansions which usually

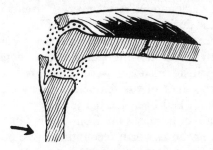

FIG. 56

Illustrating the significance of fracture of the patella, which may occur if violent flexion force is applied to a stiff knee after a fracture of the femur. The ' master' adhesions in the extensor apparatus must offer greater resistance to flexion than the intra-articular adhesions, which are readily overcome, once the extensor expansion has ruptured.

become thickened and indurated. After division of these extra-articular structures the knee can be flexed with the application of moderate force and without fracture of the patella which otherwise would occur. The best results from this operation are those where the fracture has been in the distal third of the shaft and in cases where the thigh muscles can be felt to tighten on passive flexion; old compound fractures in the lower third with adherent skin scars are particularly gratifying.

6. THE RESULTS OF PLATING OPERATIONS

Generally speaking the results of knee movement after plating the fractured femur are disappointing and this is particularly so when two plates are used for additional strength; immediately following the operation the promise of early return of knee function is usually encouraging, but at the end of one year considerable limitation of flexion is often still present. Most surgeons attribute this to adhesion of the muscle in the region of the plate; this is supported by the perfection of knee movement which results from treatment with the intramedullary nail of Kuntscher, especially when the postero-lateral approach to the shaft is used: by this method the quadriceps is scarcely touched. Experience has shown that the Henry approach, which goes through the important sliding portion of the vastus intermedius on the front of the femoral shaft, greatly retards the return of knee flexion and should be avoided at all costs.

RECOVERY OF KNEE MOTION AND THE SPEED OF UNION

Of all the factors which might affect the recovery of knee movement after a fracture of the femur *probably the most significant relates to the speed of union.* Clinical experience suggests that if bony union takes place promptly a full return of knee movement will result whether the knee was fixed throughout treatment or not; *per contra*, if delayed union occurs it is probable that some permanent restriction of knee movement will result even if strenuous attempts are made to prevent it by movement during the early stages of treatment.

The relation between early knee movement, early bone union, and final knee range is illustrated by the following personal anecdote. During the 1939-45 war five repatriated British prisoners were transferred to the author's care with gunshot fractures of the shaft of the femur caused by clean through-and-through bullet wounds. They all had been treated initially in enemy hands by a method entailing the minimum of supervision from their captors, yet the final results were so good that the lesson is worth recounting. We ourselves at this time were using a method involving a vast expenditure of energy and diligence directed to starting knee movement as soon as possible after eight weeks and at the same time striving to avoid the hazards of re-fracture. The method used on these five repatriated soldiers, on the other hand, had been : (1) four weeks of continuous skeletal traction applied through a supracondylar nail, (2) the application of a hip-spica with the traction *in situ*, (3) extraction of the supracondylar nail after hardening of the cast, and (4) no further attention until repatriated. When the plasters were removed by the writer at twelve weeks all fractures were soundly united ; knee movement recovered slowly and continuously until practically a full range was eventually obtained. Within four weeks of removal of their plasters their knee range had caught up with that of their fellows who had been the subject of overwhelming diligence and earlier knee movement. From this and other observations I believe that this would be a common experience if controlled observations could be made and provided that sound bony union occurs from the start. It is perhaps significant that despite the fact that no knee movement was possible for three months, *the patients were all taught to contract their quadriceps muscles inside the plaster casts* and, having nothing else to do and feeling that it was the only way in which they might help themselves, they obeyed their instructions implicitly.

The diagram (Fig. 57) was obtained from a series of thirty-four fractures of the femur which were free from sepsis four weeks after injury (in those cases which were compound), which involved the middle and lower thirds only, and which were in patients between twenty and forty-five years of age. Knee movement was not started until clinical union was detected. Those patients who showed clinical union *at* or *before* eight weeks (average time 6·8 weeks) had an average range of motion in the knee of 114 degrees at six months after the injury, while those not showing clinical union till *after* eight weeks (average time fifteen weeks) had 74·5 degrees of knee motion (a difference of 39·5 degrees). One year after fracture this difference in range had become less obvious and was respectively 129 degrees and 113·5 degrees (a difference of only 15·5 degrees).

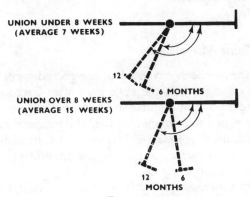

FIG. 57

Range of knee movement at six and at twelve months after fracture of the femur in relation to clinical union.

The recovery of the *last few degrees* of full knee flexion obviously cannot be dependent on simple mechanical factors *during early treatment*. The full recovery of knee motion depends on the complete recovery of elasticity in the

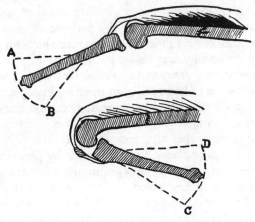

FIG. 58

Mechanical exercise over the arc BA at or before six weeks can have no direct influence on the final recovery of the range in the arc DC some six months later. Recovery of the range DC is dependent upon biological factors at the fracture site, which determine whether the provisional callus is absorbed completely or leaves permanent scar tissue in the muscle.

quadriceps muscle; this must depend on the complete resorption of all scar tissue near the site of the fracture. *It is difficult to see how exercise of the knee during the first few weeks, centred as it is on the semi-extended position (Fig. 58), can have much direct influence on the return of the last few degrees in the position of full flexion some nine months later.* The production of scar tissue round a fracture is dependent on biological factors and is the response of these tissues when bony callus is defective.

A Hypothesis of Joint Movement

Sufficient evidence has been advanced in the preceding paragraphs concerning the special instance of stiffness in the knee joint after fracture of the shaft of the femur to warrant the making of a tentative hypothesis.

It would appear reasonable to suggest that the ultimate range of joint motion depends upon two factors : *a mechanical factor* related to mobilisation by physical processes, and a *biological factor* relating to the amount of scar tissue produced in an associated muscle group.

The nature of this *mechanical* factor is obvious ; it is the freeing of muscle from involvement in callus by simple mechanical movement. But some other factor must be present in addition to the simple mechanical factor, because early movement does not always result in a perfect joint and, on the other hand, late activity can often produce a mobile joint. The *biological* factor concerns the complete absorption and removal of the temporary tissues of repair. In some cases the temporary tissue of repair is converted into permanent fibrous scar tissue which causes tethering of the surrounding muscles. Scar tissue almost invariably follows when there has been sepsis, but the healing of a closed fracture should leave no permanent scar tissue. When delayed union is present the enormous production of fibrous tissue in the periosteum is well known ; normal healing of a fracture does not result in any permanent thickening of the periosteum. The involvement of muscle by scar tissue is shown in Fig. 59, A and B.

It has been the writer's frequent observation that when a fracture of the femur reveals a noticeable absence of bony callus in the roentgenogram at about six weeks, there will always be a threat of limited knee motion, and this will remain even if the femur is treated on an apparatus permitting knee exercise. This observation is interpreted as indicating that the provisional callus, failing to become bony callus, is attempting to effect a union of the femur by permanent scar tissue and, in so doing, involves the adjacent muscles in the adhesive process. The production of large amounts of permanent scar tissue around closed fractures will only be explained when the intimate nature of delayed union is understood.

By contrast, it has been the constant observation of the writer that fractures of the femur which show plentiful bony callus, appearing at three to four weeks, will unite early, and that eventually there will be perfect motion of the knee. Profuse bony callus appears to result in less adhesion of the quadriceps than the scar tissue which, though it is radiotranslucent, we know to be present if bony callus is deficient. The profuse callus of the fractured femurs in Fig. 9B, p. 8, and Fig. 20A, p. 19, did not impair the return of full knee movement.

When fibrous tissue is produced in the tissues surrounding a closed fracture it is possible that the liberation of muscle fibres by mechanical movement is

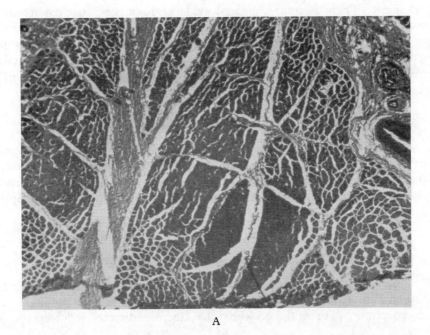

A

B

FIG. 59

A, Showing comparatively normal muscle in the vicinity of fibrous tissue round a fracture of the femoral shaft which is the site of delayed consolidation. Even here there is an excess of scar tissue in comparison with healthy muscle.

B, Showing scar tissue surrounding the site of delayed union in a fracture of the femoral shaft : note the bundles of muscle fibres included in it. This was not a compound fracture.

a futile hope. There is some collateral evidence to suggest that passive motion in these conditions may even be harmful, for when myositis ossificans develops near a fracture site it is well known that the best chance of securing a useful range of motion in the associated joint is by restriction of exercise. Passive movement in these cases can increase the area of the pathological process in the muscle fibres.

THE LAW OF CLOSED TREATMENT

I am tempted to suggest that these facts conceal a relation which might almost be elevated to the dignity of a natural law (the ' Law of Closed Treatment '), *i.e.*, that **after fracture of the shaft of a long bone, the associated joints will tolerate fixation for the duration of *normal* union without either permanent or significant loss of motion.**

JOINT STIFFNESS AFTER INJURIES INVOLVING JOINTS

Thus far I have considered only the causes of joint stiffness resulting from fractures at a distance from a joint. We must now examine what we know of the factors governing joint stiffness when the fracture directly involves the joint surfaces.

There is universal agreement, based on practical experience, that if a fracture involves a joint, mobilisation of the injured joint as early as possible is the only sure way of minimising permanent stiffness. While accepting this broad truth there are two important questions which demand discussion :

1. If the joint surfaces are distorted by a fracture, does the anatomical restoration of the joint by operation improve the final range of movement ?
2. Are there occasions when early mobilisation is harmful, and when a greater ultimate range will be obtained by an initial period of strict immobility ?

Is the operative restoration of joint contours essential ? It is frequently a simple matter to restore joint anatomy by arthrotomy and by fixing the fragments with one or two screws, at the same time preserving the theoretical advantage of early mobilisation. The functional results of this procedure vary considerably with different joints but, speaking generally, it is a surprising thing that the ultimate range of movement after the perfect restoration of intra-articular anatomy is frequently disappointing, whereas the rapid recovery of an effective range of movement in the presence of considerable distortion of the joint surfaces is often truly astonishing.

As a broad generalisation the attempt to reconstruct a distorted joint is less indicated in the non-weight-bearing upper extremity than it is in the weight-bearing lower extremity where later osteo-arthritic changes are more likely to develop.

The joints which most commonly suggest the need for arthrotomy when involved by fractures are the shoulder, elbow, knee, and ankle. The ankle usually gives a good result, but of course the range of movement in the normal ankle is not great. The elbow almost invariably does badly after operative treatment; that is to say, after operation it rarely recovers a significantly greater range than is possible by early movement with the fragments accepted in their displaced position. Particularly disappointing as regards the final range of movement are extensive open operations with internal fixation for Y-shaped fractures of the humerus in the adult. Eastwood (1937) examined the results of treating fourteen Y-shaped fractures of the elbow in adults by early mobilisation without any attempt to reduce the fragments. All except two of these patients returned to their original employment, and whereas an adequate range of flexion was achieved in all cases, he reported the following loss of extension:

Three cases .	. .	10 to 15 degrees.
Six cases	. .	30 to 35 degrees.
Three cases .	. .	45 to 60 degrees.

My own experience of the operative treatment of these fractures would lead me to expect the same loss of extension, even after exact restoration of anatomy. This extraordinary behaviour of the elbow is emphasised when one remembers that a limitation of extension by 45 degrees is not uncommon after injuries with little or no anatomical disturbance as judged radiologically. Limited extension of the elbow after dislocation, or after crack fractures of the head of the radius without displacement, therefore, must be from causes resident in the soft parts and capsule or ligaments more than in the configuration of the joint surfaces. The case illustrated in Fig. 60, which was treated initially in a collar and cuff for one week and thereafter by early motion, achieved an effective range of motion through 50 degrees centred on the right-angled position. I doubt whether any better range could have been achieved either by open reduction with internal fixation or after four weeks in bed with skeletal traction on the olecranon.

Operative exposures of the elbow joint in order to restore the radiological anatomy must inevitably increase the trauma to the capsule, and operation may delay the start of active mobilisation some ten to fourteen days compared with the mobilisation of a joint treated conservatively. This delaying effect of operation arises because operation is frequently not undertaken until almost a week has elapsed, at which time active mobilisation might be starting in a conservative regime. This early period may be a critical one in the start of organisation in capsular structures.

The Knee.—In its ability to recover movement after operative treatment the knee occupies an intermediate position, and though the range of movement is rarely full it differs from the elbow in that the most useful range includes the extended position; and even if no more than half the normal range is recovered the limitation of flexion beyond 90 degrees is not a severe disability provided that full extension is possible.

The Shoulder.—The shoulder frequently invites consideration of operative treatment in cases of fracture-dislocation where the separated head has been ejected from the joint, partially or completely, because there is obviously no method of getting a purchase on the proximal fragment by manipulation. The features against attempting a heroic open reduction are: (1) these fractures almost invariably occur in elderly patients, (2) even if reduced by open reduction, it is extremely difficult to fix the displaced head in the reduced position, and (3) in any

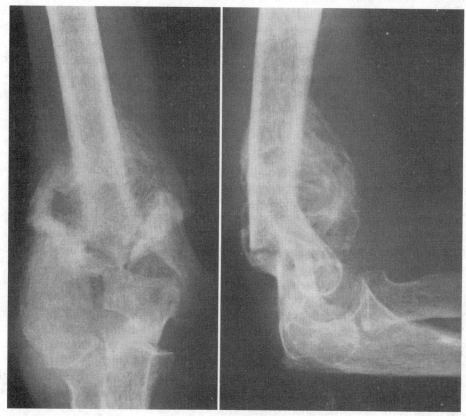

FIG. 60

T-shaped fracture treated by sling and early movement. Unlikely that accurate reduction with internal fixation would have secured a greater range than the 50 degrees which was obtained conservatively.

case the result will be almost a fibrous ankylosis of the shoulder. By early mobilisation in the displaced position sufficient movement can usually be obtained for ordinary duties below shoulder level and enough for a woman to dress her own hair (Fig. 61). Operative treatment is only indicated in these elderly patients when the humeral head is pressing on neurovascular structures in the axilla and then excision is probably the best procedure.

The Hip.—Posterior dislocations of the hip sometimes shear off a semilunar fragment of the posterior wall of the acetabulum, and though operative replacement with fixation by a screw is occasionally necessary the indications for it are rare. If a large fragment is displaced and a sciatic paralysis is present, exploration may be necessary to eliminate the possibility of compression of the nerve by the displaced fragment. In the absence of sciatic paralysis the need for exploration can be assessed on the stability of the hip after reduction ; the hip will always be stable in the fully extended position, but if when examining the supine patient under anæsthesia it falls into the dislocated position under its own weight before about 60 degrees of flexion is achieved (taking the fully extended position as zero), it would seem reasonable to advise operation.

Are there occasions when joint mobilisation can do harm ? It has long been known that the elbow frequently shows a state of 'irritability' after injury which is not seen to the same extent in any other joint. In this condition the range of elbow movement fails to increase and it may even diminish. When the extremes of the range are tested passively there is marked muscle spasm even when this spasm does not evoke pain. Deterioration of function in this way can often be traced to the patient using passive stretching movements by such exercises as carrying buckets of water in his desire to increase the mobility. In a very small percentage some ectopic ossification will be discovered in the collateral ligaments or, if the original injury was a dislocation, in the brachialis muscle. If this is discovered it is necessary to rest the elbow, but there seems to be no advantage

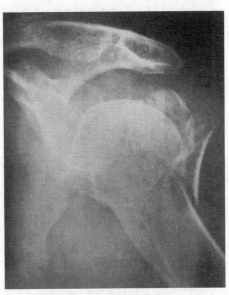

FIG. 61

Shattered fracture-subluxation of shoulder in senile patient, treated simply by early mobilisation. Patient eventually could raise hand to shoulder level without pain and with good power.

in applying a plaster cast as was often recommended in the past, and it seems sufficient merely to rest the elbow in a sling for two or three weeks before resuming active exercises again.

A puzzling thing about the persistent joint stiffness encountered in the elbow is that it is so frequently seen in children, whereas injuries involving other joints in children almost never cause lasting stiffness. If these stiff elbows are left strictly alone they will usually make a spontaneous recovery, though taking perhaps as long as two or three years before doing so. It is exceedingly unwise ever to manipulate a child's elbow to increase its range of movement. Whereas stiff elbows, occasionally, will respond dramatically to a single judicious *late* manipulation in the adult, nothing but harm can come from any attempt to increase the range of movement in a child's elbow by manipulation under anæsthesia either early or late.

An Interesting Clinical Observation.—Regarding the possible danger of excessive joint exercise, Blockey (1954) has made some interesting observations on the behaviour of the dislocated elbow which throw some light on the well-known clinical fact that passive movements are to be avoided in this condition, but that active movements can do no harm. The observation can easily be repeated on any dislocated elbow two or three weeks after reduction. At this time it will probably be found that the active and passive range of flexion and extension will

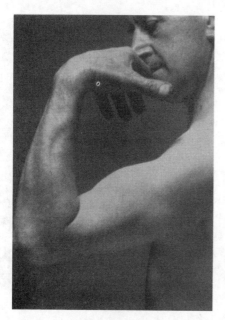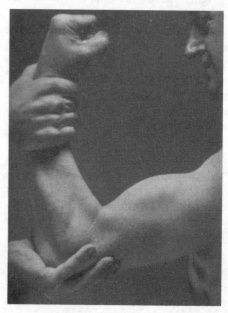

FIG. 62

Dislocated elbow fourteen days after reduction. *Left,* patient attempting maximal active flexion : note biceps brachii in only slight contraction. *Right,* patient pulling against external resistance in the mid-range of movement : note the greater tone in the biceps brachii. (*By courtesy of N. J. Blockey, F.R.C.S.*)

be through an arc of, let us say, 45 degrees centred on the 90 degrees position. If the patient is asked to pull actively against external resistance, it will be found that he can do this almost with normal power *provided that the elbow is held in the middle of the free range of movement* (*i.e.,* at 90 degrees). In this position the biceps and the brachialis muscles will be found on palpation to be in powerful contraction and the electromyograph will confirm active muscle potentials (Figs. 62, 63, 64). If, now, the external resistance is removed and the patient is asked to flex the elbow, and to hold it as strongly flexed as he possibly can, the biceps and brachialis muscles will be found to have ceased to contract, as can be proved by palpation and confirmed by the electromyograph becoming silent. It would seem reasonable to interpret this as indicating that the patient is unable to compress or stretch the organic block to flexion *because the muscles likely to do harm are inhibited as soon as the block is reached.* One presumes that the reflex mechanism permits the organic block a certain slight amount of compression or stretching but that it inhibits the source of power if it becomes excessive. It was frequently observed that this inhibition occurred even without the patient feeling pain.

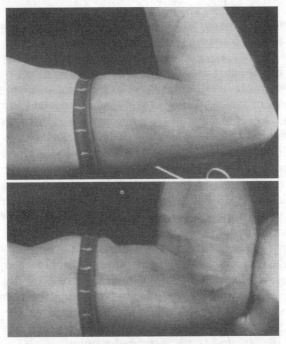

FIG. 63

Same experiment illustrated differently. Tone inhibited when contracting actively against pathological block to flexion at extreme range; tone not inhibited when contracting against external resistance in the middle range. (*By courtesy of N. J. Blockey, F.R.C.S.*)

This simple observation thus illustrates the clinical fact that repeated passive stretching, certainly in the elbow, is contrary to the natural process

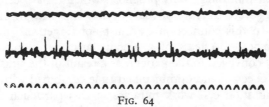

FIG. 64

Electromyograph tracings showing inhibition of action potentials in upper tracing (at extreme range of flexion), and presence of potentials in middle tracing (in middle range). (*By courtesy of N. J. Blockey, F.R.C.S.*)

of recovery of joint movement but that active mobilisation probably cannot do harm.

EXAMPLES OF FRACTURES INVOLVING JOINTS

Fractures of the Os Calcis

The treatment of this major injury is based on principles relating to (1) fractures involving joints and (2) fractures of cancellous bone.

It has been my experience that any attempt to restore the anatomical configuration of the os calcis almost invariably results in a stiff subastragaloid joint and, which is even more important, results in a painful subastragaloid joint. The striking improvement in the quality of the foot and the reduction of the time of total disablement which results from early mobilisation of the fracture in its impacted position has to be experienced to be believed and is one of the most instructive object lessons in fracture surgery.

The ill-effects on function resulting from attempts to restore the normal anatomy of the os calcis are, I believe, probably attributable to an unrecognised fibrous consolidation produced when cancellous fragments are disturbed from their natural state of intimate contact in the impacted position, and put into uncertain contact at a few precarious points in the 'reduced' position where cavities are created between the fragments filled with organising blood clot.

Powerful skeletal traction, using nails through the tibia and os calcis, as was recommended by Böhler, has been abandoned because of the universally poor results. This indicates that the advantage of restoring the normal length of the heel, which theoretically restores the normal leverage to the calf muscles, is neutralised by the disastrous effect on joint function which accompanies delayed consolidation of the os calcis in the distracted position.

Since adopting early mobilisation of the foot, without attempting to restore the anatomy of the heel, I have been impressed with the fact that most patients are able to walk with relative comfort in eight weeks, and if there is no compensation neurosis present they are capable of returning to a useful occupation nine to twelve months after the injury. In a patient who is reasonably co-operative, treated by early mobilisation, the function of the foot six months after the injury is only in the exceptional case bad enough to make one consider subastragaloid fusion.

It would appear that the gloomy prognosis which it has been customary to give the patient with a severe fracture of the os calcis is the result of 'over-treatment' of this fracture. In this connection we must not forget also the serious and far-reaching psychological ill-effects of a gloomy attitude adopted by the surgeon, and unconsciously conveyed to the patient, as a result of the sinister past reputation of this injury. A cheerful and optimistic attitude combined with early mobilisation and short hospitalisation can work miracles in this particular fracture. Even in the days when the os calcis was maltreated by distraction, and when a perpetual air of despondency surrounded the case, the very late end results (five years or more) were frequently much better than one might expect. When all compensation is settled many of these patients eventually get back to their original work.

Technical Details.—It is important to apply a firm elastic pressure dressing to the fractured os calcis and maintain this for about two weeks. Neglect to apply pressure will permit the formation of fracture blisters which may become infected. Early movements are permitted within a few days and weight-bearing encouraged after four weeks. In a few cases where there is very severe eversion of the heel an attempt may be made to manipulate and mould the heel into better shape and apply a light plaster cast, but this should not be retained for more than two or three weeks before starting mobilisation.

Fractures of the Head of the Radius

There is a wide divergence of opinion in the literature on the treatment of fractures of the head of the radius. Some surgeons advocate complete excision of the radial head whenever there is any doubt concerning the amount of displacement or comminution. I cannot help feeling that those who advocate excision of the radial head *when in doubt* do so from illogical reasoning. It is generally accepted that a fracture of the radial head is only a small part of what is a much more extensive injury to the soft tissues of the elbow joint, and that it may be the only manifestation of what has been a momentary subluxation of the elbow, sometimes accompanied by tearing of the medial collateral ligament. This is supported by the clinical fact that full extension of the elbow is always slow to return, although anatomically this movement is not related to the radial head, whereas it is common knowledge that pronation and supination almost always recover quickly and completely, yet this is the range most intimately connected with the anatomy of the radial head.

In association with a fracture of the radial head there may be a superficial contusion of the articular cartilage of the capitellum, not visible in an X-ray, and this is sometimes offered as a reason for the loss of full extension which so often follows quite a trivial crack fracture of the radial head without displacement. But superficial contusion of the cartilage covering the *capitellum* is surely no logical reason for advising excision of the *radial* head. Superficial contusion of articular cartilage is a condition ideally suitable for treatment by early joint mobilisation. Superficial contusion of the articular surface of the capitellum is unlikely to be responsible for permanent limitation of extension of the elbow, the cause of which is most probably sited in the ligaments and capsule, and excision of the radial head when in doubt will do no good to the damaged ligaments and capsule. Final proof lies in the results of excision of the radial head, and in my experience these do not show any quicker recovery of extension than in cases not operated upon. Excision of the radial head always delays early mobilisation of the injured elbow, often by as much as three weeks because, not being a true emergency, excision is often postponed one week, at which time active mobilisation would be starting in the conservative regime.

The two cases shown in Fig. 65 illustrate the above points; the patient with the almost undisplaced marginal fracture (A) had not recovered the last 30 degrees of extension five months after the injury, yet the patient with considerable comminution (B) had recovered full extension within three months. These two examples illustrate my attitude to resection of the radial head, because some surgeons would have resected the displaced and comminuted radial head in case B. As it happened, this patient had already recovered 75 per cent. of pronation and supination fourteen days after the injury, though only about 25 per cent. of the flexion-extension range had returned. With such a recovery of rotation there seemed no point in recommending excision because I did not believe that this would help the recovery of flexion and finally extension. The decision was justified by the result and she recovered full pronation and supination despite the comminution.

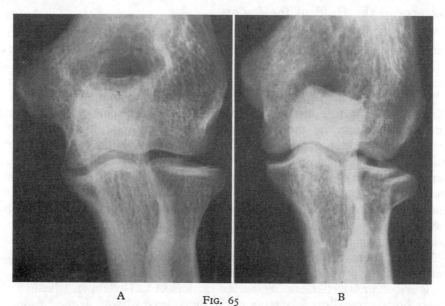

A   FIG. 65   B

Showing lack of correlation between functional result and radiological displacement in fractures of head of radius. Both cases achieved full range of pronation and supination ; case A never completely recovered full extension but case B did.

This example illustrates the importance of assessing the actual range of pronation and supination *by clinical testing* rather than by supposition from the radiological appearance.

It is sometimes suggested that if the radial head is to be excised it should be done early (*i.e.*, within the first ten days) or not at all. It is impossible to assess the necessity for excision of a radial head (which is only to restore pronation and supination) until at least two weeks have elapsed and when pain and spasm have more or less subsided. If after two weeks a comminuted fracture has not recovered an acceptable range of pronation and supination (which starts to return early if it is going to return at all) then excision can seriously be considered. I have not seen ectopic ossification follow this slightly delayed intervention.

Treatment

Patients with fractures of the radial head, even with considerable comminution, should be encouraged to practise active extension of the elbow within two or three days of the injury. They should never be allowed to retain a sling for longer than the initial week and, if possible, it should be discarded two or three days after the injury. All movements should be active and, of course, repeated passive stretching should be prohibited.

MANIPULATION OF THE ELBOW AFTER FRACTURES OF THE RADIAL HEAD

If there remains limited extension of the elbow after three months of conservative treatment of a fracture of the radial head, especially if there has been relatively little displacement, a gratifying improvement in the range of extension of the elbow can sometimes be obtained by a manipulation under anæsthesia. This is occasionally a most valuable procedure and no harm will be done if the manipulation is confined to one single occasion and is not repeated if no benefit immediately ensues.

The elbow is a joint which usually responds badly to any manipulation undertaken with the idea of improving its range of motion, and clinical teachers in the past have wisely laid great stress on condemning the practice. It must be clearly realised that I am advocating a single late manipulation in the special instance of fractures of the radial head and not for all and sundry causes of elbow stiffness after trauma and certainly never in children.

Summary of Treatment of Fractures of the Radial Head

As a working rule I would recommend the following axioms :

1. Mobilise the elbow actively as early as possible (active extension exercise after two to three days).
2. When in doubt do not excise the radial head.
3. The radial head is to be excised only if its deformity appears likely to limit pronation and supination. Practical experience shows that only very gross deformity is likely to restrict rotation.
4. Failure to recover a reasonable range of rotation by clinical testing at the end of the second week after injury, in the presence of comminution, is probably the best indication for excision of the radial head.
5. If it is decided to operate on the radial head, it should be excised *in toto*. The removal of loose fragments alone gives poor results.

REFERENCES

BLOCKEY, N. J. (1954). *J. Bone Jt Surg.* **36**, 833.
EASTWOOD, W. J. (1937). *J. Bone Jt Surg.* **19**, 364.
SCAGLIETTI, O. & CASUCCIO, C. *Estratto da La Chirurgia degli organi di movimento*, vol. xxi, Fascicolo vi, Anno 1936, xiv.
THOMPSON, T. C. (1944). *J. Bone Jt Surg.* **26**, No. 2, 366.

CHAPTER FOUR

THE TREATMENT OF FRACTURES WITHOUT
PLASTER OF PARIS

HOW often we see plaster of Paris applied merely because X-ray examination has revealed a small crack or undisplaced fracture ! On many such occasions the surgeon would probably have treated a case without plaster had he used his clinical sense alone ; he would then have been treating the injury according to his estimate of the damage inflicted on the soft parts. It is a platitude to say that soft-part injuries can be more serious than mere cracks in bone. One of the commonest instances in which the clinical assessment of an injury by soft-part damage is more important than the radiological is seen in severe ankle sprains where simple X-ray reveals ' no bone injury.' If an ankle presents very gross swelling, with extensive ecchymosis and solid induration due to the tension of the swelling, it is highly likely that there has been a rupture of the tibiofibular syndesmosis or of the external lateral ligament, and late displacement of the talus or recurrent subluxation of the ankle will occur if too early function without plaster is permitted. On the other hand, patients are frequently prevented from returning to work by plasters which are not essential but which are forced on them by surgeons who think only in terms of routine procedures and do not adjust their method to the demands of the individual problem.

It frequently happens that a surgeon is obliged to X-ray limbs for the medico-legal implication of an injury ; but the result of this examination need not make him change his clinical judgment too lightly (p. 85, Fractures of the Scaphoid). The penalty of using plaster of Paris unnecessarily when compensation is being claimed is just as serious as the danger of using too little plaster. To put an unnecessary plaster splint on a patient who has a strong compensation neurosis, or worse still, one who is wilfully exaggerating his case, is to play into the hands of a litigious patient.

A popular impulse to apply plaster to practically anything in which the X-ray shows a fracture would seem to spring from an unvoiced belief that plaster is some sort of dressing which, when applied to the skin, accelerates the healing of the underlying bone. It is as well to remember that the human species has survived in the struggle for existence by making a fair attempt to unite its own fractures during the millions of years which preceded the discovery of plaster of Paris. A critical mechanical inquiry into the motive for applying a cast will often show that the aim of ' immobilisation,' by which plaster is fondly supposed to act, often results in nothing of the kind. It is true that the liberal application of plaster to all and sundry of the minor fractures encountered in a casualty department can do no serious harm to any, and may do good to some; but there is, however, a deeper motive for criticising the too liberal use of plaster. The healing of bone and the recovery of flexibility in soft tissues are phenomena which are basic to the work of the orthopædic surgeon. To understand the materials of his trade the surgeon must observe the behaviour of these materials just as much in the untreated as in the treated case. The casualty surgeon must snatch at any opportunity which presents itself for observing how quickly the untreated Colles' fracture becomes painless and how quickly the full power of the grip returns. It is, moreover, from the behaviour of healing fractures that the basic operations or arthrodesis and bone grafting derive and from these the greater part of modern orthopædic surgery is built. It is by observing the behaviour of the 'minor' fracture that the orthopædic surgeon learns to think in terms of healing bone; if this period of his training is circumscribed by dogma and devoted purely to the execution of routines (*i.e.*, Colles', four weeks in plaster; tibias, twelve; scaphoids, six; etc.), his apprenticeship has been wasted.

PRINCIPLES IN THE TREATMENT OF FRACTURES WITHOUT FIXATION

The treatment of fractures without rigid external fixation is no new idea; the method was advocated many years ago by the French surgeon Lucas-Championnière who described in elaborate detail a system of massage for each fracture and dislocation. Many of the reasons why the method could never be popular are economic: thus it would require an enormous personnel to administer it to an industrial region and a large number of hospital beds would be required, whereas plaster fixation renders domiciliary treatment possible. At the present time the treatment of minor fractures without splintage tends to receive insufficient publicity (though most surgeons instinctively practise it when the occasion arises), and interest is aroused only when major fractures, such as those of the os calcis or the spine, are treated by early movement. Yet it is in the common, minor fracture that the advantages of abandoning external fixation are most apparent.

In the following paragraphs an attempt is made to indicate what type of fracture can be treated without plaster fixation and what general principles might guide the surgeon in choosing this treatment, but before this can be done it is first necessary to expose certain **popular misconceptions regarding plaster fixation**:

1. That the fragments of a fresh fracture are always mobile unless fixed by artificial means.
2. That a plaster cast will prevent such mobility.
3. That displacement will increase if the limb is not splinted.
4. That plaster fixation accelerates fracture healing.
5. That the quality of the end result will be better after treatment with plaster than without.

That the Fragments are Mobile if not Splinted

In the mechanics of fixation the fractured shafts of the long bones differ considerably from the short bones. Errors in the treatment of fractures of the short bones often have their origin in the application of principles which are only indicated for fractures of the long bones. When we attempt actively to elevate, without splintage, an extremity which contains a fractured long bone, movement at the fracture is produced by the weight of the distal limb acting through the leverage offered by the long fragments. In fractures involving the short bones, the length of the levers and the weight of the distal limb are both small and, unless muscular contractions generate an indirect force, there is practically no strain imposed on such fractures during gentle and restricted movements of the associated joints. Relative to their length, the short bones are of large diameter, which renders them mechanically stable when fractured, whereas the long bones, being narrow in comparison with their length, are exceedingly unstable when fractured.

In fractures through cancellous bone, impaction is common and this offers one obvious explanation of the absence of movement at a fracture when the whole limb is moved. In the long bones impaction is impossible because both fragments are of ivory bone (a fact which students often seem to overlook), but impaction of an ivory shaft can take place into the cancellous extremity of a long bone, as is commonly seen in the Colles' fracture and less commonly in necks of the femur and humerus.

In the miniature long bone—the metacarpals and metatarsals—isolated fractures are splinted by the adjacent bones through the strong interosseous ligaments which bind them together.

Fractures of cancellous and cortical bone differ considerably in their rate of healing. Whereas a fracture in the shaft of a long bone may be mobile for six weeks (because of the great leverage on the fracture site and scanty callus), a fracture in cancellous bone may be clinically firm in this time though it would of course be unfit to bear weight until true consolidation had occurred.

In recent fractures it seems reasonable to interpret pain on the movement of adjacent joints as a sign that the fracture is being disturbed. That the pain in a recent fracture does in fact come from the fracture itself is shown by the absence of pain when local anæsthesia is introduced into a fracture hæmatoma. Therefore it can be considered as an axiom that, in a recent fracture, as long as a range of movement is possible in neighbouring joints without evoking pain in a healing fracture, no significant movement is taking place at the fracture site; **significant movement at a fresh fracture is threatened only when the painless range is exceeded.**

That a Plaster of Paris Splint prevents Movement in a Fracture

Perkins has attempted to rationalise the teaching of fracture treatment by dividing the functions of splints into two types; these serve the functions respectively of ' simple splintage ' and ' immobilisation.' The *simple splint* is capable only of controlling gross external deformity of the limb as a whole; that is to say, it will hold the fragments in alignment while healing is taking place, and will result in the restoration of the normal external shape to the body. The function of *immobilisation*, on the other hand, implies the absolute abolition of microscopic movement between the bone ends during the process of healing. It is obvious that there is no method of external splintage which could fulfil this definition of immobilisation, and therefore some form of internal fixation by a metal splint or bone graft is the only perfect means of enforcing it. Even in fractures of the carpal scaphoid it is doubtful whether the most skilfully applied plaster splint can immobilise the fragments, because of the movement which is possible between the skin and bones. Similar reflection will show how futile it is to expect a walking plaster to immobilise a fracture in the tarsus or metatarsus; at every step of the foot the soft cushion of tissues in the sole of the foot is compressed and the arches of the foot deflect under the body weight and spring back again when the weight is relieved (Fig. 66). A walking plaster for such fractures is actually no more effective than a leather boot. In recent fractures of the forefoot treated in a walking plaster the patient invariably walks with weight on his heel

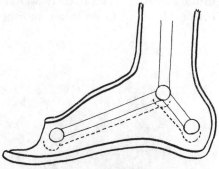

FIG. 66

Diagram illustrating futility of the idea that a walking plaster can immobilise the tarsus. Under body weight the arches of the foot deflect and the soft tissues in the sole of the foot are compressed whether the limb is in plaster or not.

during the first week or two; only when healing is moderately advanced does he permit the forefoot to exert any pressure on the sole of the plaster. In Fig. 67 is seen a fracture of the first metatarsal treated by this method; the patient was walking in a boot and without pain by the fourth week and was back at work in six weeks.

That the Displacement will Increase if not Splinted

On viewing the X-ray of a recent fracture there is often a subconscious fear that the deformity will increase unless a plaster is applied. A spontaneous increase in deformity is inevitable if fractures of the shafts of the long bones are left without artificial support, because the leverage of long fragments alters the displacement at every change in the patient's posture by reason of the heavy weight of the distal limb. But this is not true of many of the smaller fractures; **in fractures of the short bones the displacement is limited by the extent to which the tough fibrous elements in the vicinity have been torn.** It is thus unlikely that a displaced fracture of a short bone will move beyond the initial position of displacement unless further violence is used to rupture more fibrous tissue.

83

There is one important exception to this statement, mentioned on page 32. There is always the possibility that what may be diagnosed as an 'undisplaced' fracture, judged by the initial radiograph, may have been grossly displaced at the moment of the injury and in the process of first-aid splintage may have been reduced into almost perfect position. Subsequent displacement, as a result of ligaments and soft parts being torn, may later take the surgeon by surprise. This accident is a trap for the unwary in the case of the ankle fractures. It is very unlikely that a bi-malleolar fracture could have been sustained without considerable tearing of soft parts, so beware the diagnosis of 'undisplaced' fractures if bi-malleolar, because if early weight-bearing in plaster is permitted (which is a reasonable thing to do in an undisplaced fracture) it is probable that the original

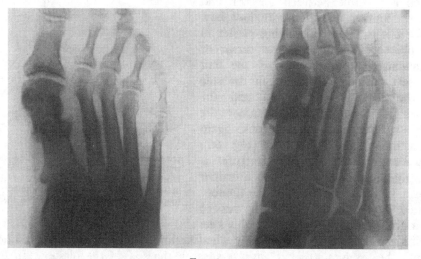

FIG. 67

Fractures of the shaft of the first and second metatarsals treated without plaster of Paris. By walking on his heel this patient was able to keep on his feet and was back at light work in six weeks.

deformity will develop. This accident is especially likely to catch the unwary surgeon because one does not usually insist on repeated radiographic checks of the position when the original diagnosis is an undisplaced fracture, and thus the first intimation of displacement may be when the plaster is finally removed.

When a fracture has been reduced by manipulation it will always be necessary to apply a splint to prevent recurrence of the initial displacement; but **if an attempt at reduction fails and the position is thereby not improved, splintage is no longer essential** and treatment by early movement may then offer certain advantages.

That Plaster Fixation will Speed Healing

Prompting the application of many plasters is the fear that a fracture may fail to unite unless it is splinted. The fear of pseudarthrosis is often quite unfounded and often arises by loose inference from isolated cases which are erroneously regarded as instances of a general principle. In fractures of the long bones some form of external fixation is absolutely essential in order to restrict gross movement, but these factors are absent in the short and the miniature long bones and therefore in these it is to be expected that healing might proceed without external fixation. There are two notable exceptions to this statement, namely : fractures of the carpal scaphoid and of the neck of the femur. The specific nature of these two examples is shown by the fact that they should be further particularised into fractures of the *waist* and *proximal pole* of the scaphoid, and of the *midcervical* and *subcapital* region of the femoral neck. The common factor which isolates this small group from fractures of the rest of the skeleton is the complication of *ischæmic necrosis*. It cannot be too strongly insisted that ischæmic necrosis is a *complication* of fracture repair and that the study of fracture healing must not include such instances in the healing of ' normal ' fractures. The disaster of pseudarthrosis which follows the treatment of a fracture of the carpal scaphoid by early mobilisation is so well known that it is not surprising it should influence the treatment of other injuries. There is, however, no logical reason why fractures of the cuneiform, os magnum, or tubercle of the scaphoid should be treated by rigid external fixation. It is possible that further study may show that ischæmia is a factor in all fractures where slow union is common, but for practical purposes the condition of ischæmic necrosis is to be regarded as a complication only encountered in a few well-known sites, such as the talus, the medial malleolus, dislocations of the semilunar, dislocation of the hip, and sometimes in the distal thirds of the shaft of the tibia and of the ulna.

As regards the effect of plaster fixation on the speed of fracture healing, it hardly needs to be pointed out that plaster cannot *accelerate* healing ; plaster merely ensures that the limb will be in good alignment when healing has taken place. The rate of healing is a function of the activity of the osteoblast and in all probability healing takes place, under normal conditions, according to certain time phases related to various chemical and physical changes. But though these processes cannot be accelerated they can easily be inhibited by unfavourable external conditions ; the final stages of ossification can be delayed by faulty blood supply or by gross and continuous movement. **The aim of fracture treatment is to eliminate all deleterious influences rather than to accelerate union.**

That the Quality of the Result is Better after Plaster Treatment than Without

This belief arose from the teaching of Böhler who taught that by applying plaster to enable the splinted limb to be used, static muscular contractions would maintain the blood supply and thereby accelerate union. Böhler believed that by preventing ' intercellular œdema ' the stiffening of joint capsules as the cause of permanent stiffness would be eliminated. Though containing much truth the result of this dogma has not supported his claims ; delayed union of the tibia still remains a common occurrence, joint stiffness occurs as often as after any other method, and late œdema is a frequent complication following removal of the plaster splint.

But apart from theoretical matters one must face a practical question. Can any significant saving of time be effected in treating fractures without plaster? In the upper extremity there is no doubt that some saving of time is possible by treating suitable fractures without plaster, and that the patient, particularly if a professional man, may find the convalescence more tolerable without plaster (*i.e.*, facilities for washing and being normally clothed, etc.). In the lower extremity, however, the saving of time is less significant. Many small fractures (as, for instance, an undisplaced fracture of an external malleolus) may be completely rehabilitated within four weeks if treated in a flexible dressing, but against this is the fact that the patient may be totally incapacitated from work for the first two weeks, whereas in plaster he may be ambulant earlier though with a slightly longer overall disability.

CASES SUITABLE FOR TREATMENT WITHOUT PLASTER

The following list comprises those fractures which are suited to early mobilisation without plaster fixation :

Shafts of fibula.	Olecranon (if undisplaced).
Tarsal bones.	Patella (if stellate or transverse without
Metatarsals.	separation).
' March ' fractures.	Elbow fractures.
Styloid process of fifth metatarsal.	Tuberosity of carpal scaphoid.
Phalanges of toes.	Other carpal bones (excluding waist of
Metacarpals.	scaphoid).
Os calcis.	Mild compression fractures lumbar spine.
Tibial condyles (in the aged).	Pelvis.
Thoracic spine.	Central dislocation of the hip.

POSITIVE INDICATIONS FOR PLASTER FIXATION

To contrast with the preceding list of fractures suitable for treatment by early movement, the *positive indications for the treatment of fractures by plaster* might be stated in the following terms :

1. To maintain a position secured by reduction.
2. To ' immobilise ' if movement is likely when adjacent joints are moved.
3. To ' immobilise ' when one fragment is prone to ischæmic necrosis.
4. To permit weight-bearing in order to stimulate bony union in delayed union of long bones.
5. For economic reasons, *i.e.*, to evacuate hospital beds or make a patient ambulant for his personal convenience.

THE PRESSURE BANDAGE

In the treatment of simple fractures without plaster of Paris the application of a well-designed and well-applied pressure dressing often does not receive the attention which its importance merits. A carefully applied pressure dressing can provide some degree of *splintage by reason of its rigidity* and yet at the same time allow of *movement through a restricted range*. The efficacy of bandaging painful joints is well known in veterinary practice and the methods of the hunting field which can keep a horse at work with knees and fetlocks bandaged can be applied equally well to the rider.

The most highly organised example of the semi-flexible pressure dressing is that applicable to the knee and often referred to as the ' Robert Jones bandage ' (Fig. 68). It consists of three layers of wool and three layers of domette bandage. The layers are put on gently but firmly and the whole bandage extends some

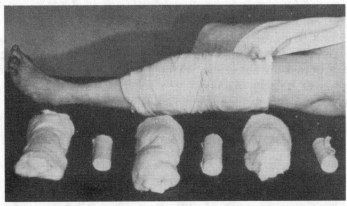

FIG. 68

Robert Jones pressure bandage. Final bandage extends from the mid-calf to mid-thigh, is 2 inches in thickness, and its special features are : local support from its turgidity, control of swelling by its pressure, and slight movement by its trace of flexibility.

6 inches above and below the joint and attains a thickness of about 2 inches. By reaching well down the calf the troublesome swelling of the calf, with painful cutting in of the bandage which results with short knee bandages, is prevented. In this connection it is worth noting that adhesive strapping applied as a pressure dressing to a knee is a most unsuitable and most uncomfortable dressing, and should be avoided at all costs. By reason of its bulk the Jones bandage provides an effective check to movement of more than about 10 degrees.

This type of dressing for the majority of knee injuries is infinitely better than any form of plaster cast ; **a plaster is incapable of applying continuous gentle pressure once an effusion has started to diminish.** As soon as the efficacy of this simple but highly scientific dressing is appreciated it will be found that **very few plaster cylinders need be used for the non-operative treatment of knee injuries or fractures of the patella.**

CHAPTER FIVE

PLASTER TECHNIQUE

MANY failures in conservative treatment can be traced to inadequate plaster technique. A good manipulative reduction is often allowed to slip during the clumsy application of plaster. The surgeon who aspires to skill in the conservative method must subject himself to a long apprenticeship in ' plastercraft.' Skill is not to be learned from books but only by continuous repetition for at least one year, and the casualty officer who regards the application of plasters as a menial task to be delegated to juniors or to the nursing staff will be well advised to transfer his attention to another specialty. Until the surgeon's hands have acquired an automatic rhythm, being able to pass and mould the turns of bandages quickly, regularly, and subconsciously, his mind is not free to devote its entire concentration to the tissues of the fracture.

PADDED AND UNPADDED PLASTERS

Plaster casts can be divided into three types : (1) ' badly padded ' plaster, (2) unpadded plaster, and (3) padded plaster.

' Badly Padded ' Plaster

It was against the background of the badly padded plaster that Böhler inveighed with such effect, and it was Böhler's teaching which established the use of the unpadded plaster, applied directly to the skin without any soft material intervening. So powerful were his convictions that even now the word padding is still regarded in many circles as something unmentionable or as something for which to apologise. It will later be seen that in this book the skin-tight plaster is not recommended for general use ; I believe that when properly applied the padded plaster is just as efficient as an unpadded one, is much more comfortable, and has certain subtle advantages.

The badly padded plaster can be quickly dismissed ; it is loose on the limb and cannot therefore fix the fragments. **Unless the surgeon pays extreme attention to detail in using padding correctly he will produce a badly padded plaster before he realises it.**

Unpadded Plaster

This type of plaster is made by applying the turns of wet bandage directly to the skin without the intervention of any textile. The closeness of its application to the limb, and to some extent the actual adhesion to the skin, is believed by some to enhance the fixation of a fracture. In Böhler's original technique not even stockinet was allowed between plaster and skin. Even if stockinet is used the plaster which results can still be regarded, for all practical purposes, as an unpadded cast.

Provided that certain elementary points in technique are observed there is no danger in the skin-tight plaster. It is important that the bandage should never be pulled tight, as when applying an ordinary cotton bandage to hold on a dressing. In the unpadded technique the bandage should be made to *roll itself round the limb*. By laying the wet roll of plaster on the skin and pushing it round the curves of the limb with the flat of the hand it will be made to find its own way without causing tight ridges. In no circumstances should the roll of plaster be lifted off the limb and pulled. The technique is one which is quite easily learned, though like any technique it takes many months to acquire sufficient skill to produce a masterly finish. *This technique is considerably easier to acquire than is the padded plaster technique.*

Though the padded plaster is the one which the writer recommends for general use there are at least three conditions where the unpadded plaster is essential: (1) all plaster strips or slabs should be applied direct to the skin (as in the Colles' fracture) and (2) the scaphoid of the wrist; and (3) the Bennett's fracture should always be treated in unpadded plasters.

Padded Plaster

The real merits of a padded plaster cannot be appreciated until good examples of the technique are examined. My own interest in this type of cast was first stimulated by examining the work of visitors to Britain trained in the Bologna School (Morandi, 1948).

In this method a layer of cotton-wool is interposed between the skin and the plaster, which is then firmly compressed against the limb by applying the wet plaster bandage *under tension*. Instead of the wool rendering the plaster loose, **the elastic pressure of the wool actually enhances the fixation of the limb by compensating for slight shrinkage in the tissues after application of the cast.** The amount of tension used in pulling tight the individual turns of plaster is difficult to describe; it can be surprisingly high and yet it never appears to cause any embarrassment to the circulation. When expertly applied I feel quite sure that these plasters grip the limb more firmly and keep this grip for a longer time than do skin-tight plasters. I have often heard intelligent patients, treated in a so-called skin-tight plaster for fractures of the tibia, say that their legs were quite loose inside their plasters on getting up in the morning, and that they could only bear weight with comfort when their legs had again swollen to fit the plaster tightly.

In the padded plaster technique the cotton-wool is carefully applied as an even layer of rolled wadding. Depending on the thickness of the wadding, sufficient turns should be applied to build up a layer of loose wadding measuring about half an inch in thickness which will later be compressed by the overlying plaster to about an eighth of an inch. **The care with which this layer of wool is applied is essential for success; it must not obscure the shape of the limb by being put on in careless and ugly lumps.** The sheet wadding, if it is not already rolled, should be carefully prepared in rolls before application.

In applying the plaster the method of applying tension is difficult to describe; the action of putting on each turn lies half-way between an ordinary bandaging movement in which the roll is lifted off the limb, pulled, and 4 or 5 inches of

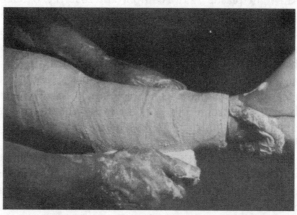

A

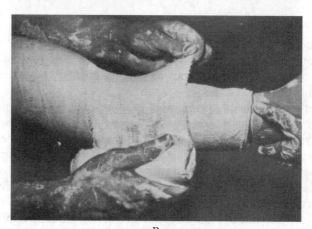

B

FIG. 69
Method of applying plaster bandage over padding.
A, Applying tension to the bandage by pressure of the thenar eminence exerted in the middle of the bandage so as to avoid cutting-in of the edges.
B, Making a tuck to accommodate the tapering limb.

stretched bandage then wound round the limb, and the unpadded technique where the roll of bandage lies continuously in contact with the limb. The roll of bandage remains in contact with the surface of the limb almost continuously but instead of being lightly guided round the limb it is *pressed* and *pushed* round the limb by the pressure of the thenar eminence under a strong pushing force directed in the length of the surgeon's forearm. The technique is illustrated in Fig. 69, A. It will be seen that pressure is applied through the surgeon's thenar eminence at the middle of the width of the bandage so that no excess of pressure can fall on either edge of the bandage and so cause a sharp ridge. Each turn is applied slowly and is settled carefully in position, the surgeon's hands following the natural inclination of the bandage without forcing it unduly in any uneasy direction. At tapering parts of the limb the turns are made to lie evenly by small tucks, made with a quick movement of the index finger of the left hand before each turn is smoothed into position (Fig. 69, B). *The durability of the cast and its strength for a given lightness depend on the welding together of the individual turns by these smoothing movements of the left hand*; it is erroneous to imagine that the first and the last layers are the only ones which need to be applied carefully; every layer must be applied with equal deliberation.

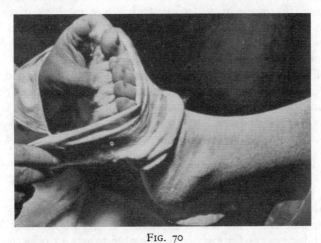

FIG. 70

Technique of applying plaster at the toes. Each toe is wrapped with a twist of wool and then all together in a turn of sheet wadding. The plaster is applied over the toes and then cut back to the desired level. By this means adequate space is left for movement of the digits. (*Dr Casuccio.*)

It will be seen from the above description that this technique precludes the use of plaster slabs; the whole cast is built up from circular bandages.

In applying the bandage it is difficult to advise as to how much tension must be used. It is surprising how much tension can be tolerated if it is evenly distributed over a large surface area; I have never yet applied one of these plasters too tightly. In below-knee plasters it is important that the bandage should be pulled very tight indeed in the proximal part because, unless the wool and the soft muscles are both powerfully compressed, it will be found that the plaster when completed will be as loose as a Wellington boot; in the distal part of the plaster round the ankle the tension must be less, but even so it must be enough to make the wool spring at each turn of the bandage.

In Fig. 70 is shown a method of padding each toe separately with a wisp of wool; this enables the toes to have freedom of movement when the wool is picked out after hardening of the plaster.

' End-to-end Rhythm '

The hall-mark of a good plaster is that it should be of even thickness from end to end. It is only too common to find plasters, such as those for the scaphoid or the Pott's fractures, which exceed even half an inch in thickness at the wrist or ankle and yet taper away to one layer of bandage at the upper and lower apertures (Fig. 71). These plasters are not criticised on æsthetic grounds alone but because they fail to fix the fragments by being functionally too short. If the lower aperture of a forearm plaster is too thin the accurate modelling of the plaster to the palmar creases is valueless, and movement of the wrist becomes possible through a considerable range.

The cast which tapers in thickness towards each end results from the surgeon being *obsessed by the region of the injury* and failing to think of the plaster as a whole. A cast of even thickness throughout is more easily produced if the bandage is applied without thinking about the site of the injury and *by deliberately concentrating on making the two ends of the cast of adequate thickness*. The surgeon should discipline himself **never to apply two turns in the same place except at the ends ;** this can be done by establishing a progressive ' backward and forward rhythm ' from the top to the bottom of the plaster (Fig. 72).

Quick-setting and Slow-setting Plaster

Since the publication of the early editions of this book the manufacturers of proprietary plaster bandages produce grades which are very satisfactory and which do not set too quickly.

It is an essential point in plaster technique that the first bandage to be applied should still be soft when the last is finished. If the plaster is soft the surgeon can feel a mobile fracture through it and be able to mould it as he wishes. **One of the commonest causes of defective reduction is that the plaster is allowed to reach the consistency of wet cardboard before the final turn has been applied ;** the surgeon is then unable to feel any movement of the reduction which he is striving to secure. When using the padded plaster technique, with its deliberate passage of each turn under tension, the use of quick-setting plaster is a serious mistake because this kind of plaster always takes a little longer to apply than the unpadded cast.

One of the commonest causes of premature setting, due to slow application of the plaster, is a tendency to use a large number of narrow bandages. While there are rare occasions when 4-inch bandages may be needed, I strongly recommend that the 6-inch and 8-inch bandages should be regarded as the standard size for anything except fingers. The 6-inch bandage should be used for the forearm and the 8-inch bandage for the ankle. Many surgeons only think of the 8-inch bandage when plaster jackets or hip-spicas are in mind.

The importance of infrequent plaster changing needs repeated emphasis. The ill effects of changing plasters in precipitating delayed union makes all the more obvious the importance of a skilful plaster technique. **A cast should never be applied carelessly with the thought in the surgeon's mind that**

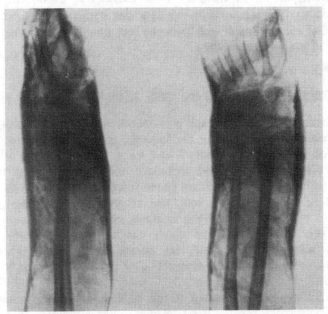

FIG. 71

A badly applied plaster. The surgeon has been obsessed by the level of the injury; the effective length of the cast is too short because the upper and lower limits are thin and ill-defined.

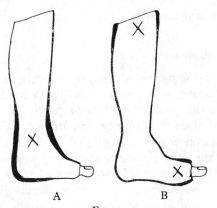

A   B

FIG. 72

A, By concentrating too much on the site of the fracture there is a tendency to produce a thick plaster with thin extremities.

B, By concentrating on the extremities of the plaster the site of the fracture will generally look after itself, and a light rigid cast will be obtained of equal thickness throughout. In this method no two turns of plaster are ever applied in the same place except at the extremities (the ' backward and forward rhythm ').

it can be changed 'next month' if it turns out to be imperfect; the surgeon should apply a plaster with the idea that it might be made to last for the whole period of the treatment and with the full intention that when it comes off the patient will not require another.

THE TRIPLE SEQUENCE IN THE APPLICATION OF PLASTER

The application of plaster must now be considered in an actual reduction. There is a great difference between the leisurely application of plaster to a healing fracture which is clinically 'sticky' and to a recent fracture with a mobile deformity. Without a rehearsed technique the reduction and fixation of a mobile fracture is often a hectic and nerve-wracking business with surgeon and assistant getting in each other's way, the surgeon impeding the application of the plaster by the assistant and the assistant obstructing the reduction by the surgeon. Even if the reduction turns out to be satisfactory under these conditions it will often be found, on examining the finished cast, that the position of the joints may not be that for ideal function (*i.e.*, the foot may be in equinus, etc.).

These difficulties are eliminated if the process of reduction and fixation is regarded as possessing *three distinct phases*. These phases, though generally applicable, are seen at their best in the reduction and fixation of a Pott's or Bennett's fracture.

Phase 1. Examination and rehearsal.
Phase 2. Plastering.
Phase 3. Reduction and holding.

1. Examination and Rehearsal

The first phase of the sequence is given up entirely to an examination of the displacement and to making an assessment of the forces required to reduce and hold the reduction. In this phase the **effect of gravity** on the displacement must be remembered, as it is often of very great importance. The position of the limb must be discovered which makes use of gravity in holding the reduction or, alternatively, the position must be found where any undesirable effects of gravity can be eliminated. The **amount of force** needed to correct the displacement must be assessed and the **range of excursion** from the position of greatest deformity to the position of apparent reduction must be committed to memory. Sometimes it will be found that the reduction can be held by a minimum force applied at a key point; in this case the **key point** must be localised for future reference.

The examination and rehearsal is not complete until the surgeon is sure that he can reduce the fracture with one or, at the most, two purposive movements and hold it in reduction without persistent and indecisive 'fiddling' movements of his hands.

2. Plastering

With the knowledge gained from the previous phase placed temporarily on one side the plaster must now be applied. To do this the limb is held by the assistant in the position of approximate reduction. It is my belief that the surgeon himself should apply the plaster because the surgeon alone appreciates the urgency of the situation. The quick application of plaster must not be impeded by attempts to hold a precise reduction. The cast is applied as quickly as possible, so that it is still completely soft by the time the last turn is applied. A slow-setting plaster is necessary for this purpose; if the cast is a large one, the final touches should not be added at this stage—at this stage only sufficient plaster should be applied to hold the reduced position temporarily; the plaster can later be made thicker and completed at its upper and lower limits.

3. Reduction and Holding

Sufficient plaster having been applied just to hold the fracture when set, the surgeon now takes the limb from the assistant and prepares to apply the rehearsed movement of reduction. With the plaster wet and soft he should be able to recognise clearly the sensation of reduction which he learned in Phase 1, though now it will be rather muffled by the intervening plaster and wool. Having applied the rehearsed movements of reduction he holds on, without further agitation of his hands, until the cast has set. During the last few minutes of the setting he can move his hands a little to obliterate any abrupt local impression which might invite a pressure sore. The cast is now completed to the required final thickness and the upper and lower limits shaped to limits appropriate to the case.

FUNCTION WHILE IN PLASTER

In promoting function while in plaster a simple clinical fact needs mention because it is often overlooked; perhaps it is overlooked because it is so obvious. **When the decision is made to remove a plaster it is unwise to do so if the patient is not by this time already capable of good function in the plaster.** Thus in the case of a Pott's fracture at ten weeks, it is unwise to remove the plaster if the patient is walking badly or walking only with the assistance of a stick. If the plaster is taken off at this stage it will be found in all probability that the patient may need two sticks, or even be unable to walk at all. If a patient is walking badly, and needing a great deal of assistance from a stick, the reason should have been discovered and put right long before the calendar time for removal of the plaster has arrived. There are three common causes of defective function in a walking plaster :

1. *An Uncomfortable Plaster or Bad Walking Heel.*—The plaster may have been uncomfortable for weeks as a result of being badly applied; the patient often thinks that pain is to be expected from a fracture and does not report it. **If the plaster is a bad one, the patient may never be able to learn to walk while he is in the cast.**

95

2. *Failure of Psychic Rehabilitation.*—The patient may not have received the encouragement necessary to show him that he *can* walk ; he may never have seen other patients in the same type of splint playing games or exhibiting some similar example of robust function. The importance of a **cheerful rehabilitation service in close contact with the surgeon cannot be over-emphasised ; it should never be a separate service in a general hospital with divided loyalty to a separate director.**

3. *Bone Atrophy.*—Post-traumatic osteodystrophy is an obscure but fortunately rare condition. In these cases, after removal of plaster, the limb swells and may become even more painful than before. It is my present opinion that these cases are best left in plaster for a very long time, and certainly left until good function has been obtained while still in plaster. Fortunately these cases are rare ; the more expert the fracture team the less frequently they are seen : an observation which tends to suggest that they are possibly the result of treatment in plasters which have been too tight or plasters which have been painful for many weeks and have induced a superadded hysterical state of disuse. The condition is rarely seen in the phlegmatic type of patient who is unafraid of his injury and who has confidence in his surgeon.

ERRORS IN APPLYING THE PADDED CAST

1. Attempting to plaster at the same time as attempting to hold a precise reduction.
2. Applying wool carelessly and in shapeless lumps instead of having it previously neatly prepared in rolls and bandaging it on with very great care to give an even layer.
3. Not bandaging tightly enough, with the result that the finished plaster is loose.
4. Not bandaging the fleshy proximal part with greater tension than in the bony distal part, resulting in a below-knee plaster of the ' Wellington boot ' effect.
5. Failing to recognise the sensation of reduction through plaster, as a result of using quick-setting plaster which becomes stiff too quickly.
6. Failing to recognise the sensation of reduction, from inadequate examination during the initial phase of reduction.
7. Applying the plaster carelessly on the supposition that there is no harm in changing it at any time.

Windowed Plasters

Generally speaking, the making of windows in plasters is not a policy to be encouraged. The danger of œdematous tissues herniating through a window, especially in plasters on the lower extremity, and the theories of Winnett Orr on the closed plaster treatment of osteomyelitis, have made many people regard the windowing of plasters as a surgical crime.

Provided, however, that certain technical matters are observed in nursing a windowed plaster, there are numerous occasions on which it can be used to advantage, although the advent of antibiotics has probably made even these occasions less frequent than formerly.

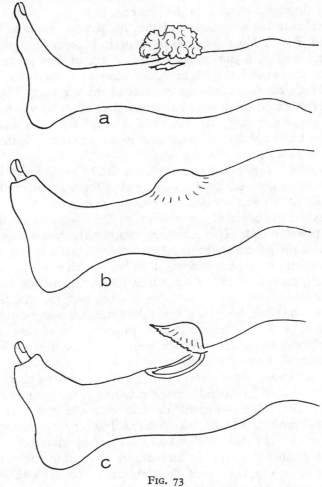

FIG. 73

Simple method of locating a window accurately over the desired point in a plaster. Firm lump of wool applied over wound (a), causes a visible bulge in the finished plaster (b), which can be cut off with a sharp knife (c).

In the recent world war it was a frequent experience to find that compound fractures discharging copious pus seemed to reach a standstill in their healing after about three months in closed plaster. Beyond this time the decomposing discharges accumulating in the plaster seemed to become irritant and caused excoriation of the surrounding skin, prevented the growth of new epithelium, and produced exuberant unhealthy granulation tissue. If the plaster was windowed

97

in this type of case, and a few daily dressings performed, a remarkable improvement in the condition of the tissues was noticeable within a few days. Similarly, in cases where a compound fracture had been grafted with pinch grafts or Thiersch grafts, in the presence of slight infection, it was found that the grafts tended to dissolve, after a preliminary 'take,' unless the graft was washed at about the fourth day through a window in the plaster.

If it is decided to use a windowed plaster, the patient should as far as possible be discouraged from holding the limb too long in a dependent position, and for this reason the method is not to be advised in ambulatory plasters. It is also important that the wound should be under pressure from a properly designed pad of wool firmly bandaged into the aperture of the window. The maintenance of this local pressure on the wound has a beneficial effect on wound healing, and it is indeed a paradox that the windowed plaster, far from causing window herniation, can be the means of enhancing local pressure over the wound in a way which is impossible in a closed plaster.

To maintain local pressure in the window a pad of wool should be built up to project, in the uncompressed state, about 2 inches above the level of the window. The pad should fit the window like a piston and not extend on to the surface of the plaster beyond the edges of the window, as this would defeat the piston-like action of the pressure pad. It is necessary to apply the bandage under sufficient pressure to cause the patient slight initial discomfort when it is first applied.

Not infrequently a surgeon may be unwilling to window a plaster if he has to do it himself, because of the labour which the cutting of the hole can entail. Even if an electric plaster saw is available it often happens that the window is made over the wrong site, and when it is fully extended to encompass the wound it has become unnecessarily large. It is an important point that *windows should be kept as small as is compatible with their purpose*, and for this reason they should be centred accurately over the discharging sinus. A useful technical hint is to apply a piece of wool—rolled firmly into a ball or sausage shape and slightly smaller than the size of the wound—over the centre of the wound before applying the plaster bandage. The result will be that when the plaster is complete the ball of wool will produce a 'bleb' situated exactly over the centre of the wound. The top of this bleb can then be sliced off with a sharp knife held parallel to the surface of the plaster and without any danger of cutting the patient. If the plaster is allowed to dry, the top of the bleb can be cut off with a saw held flat on the surface of the cast, and once the central hole has been made in the correct position it is a simple matter to enlarge it with a sharp knife (Fig. 73).

REFERENCE

MORANDI (1948). *Technica degli Apparecchi Gessati.* Bologna : Scientifiche Instituto Rizzoli.

CHAPTER SIX

FRACTURES OF THE SHAFT OF THE HUMERUS

A FRACTURE of the shaft of the humerus is perhaps the easiest of major long bones to treat by conservative methods. The humerus is a bone which generally unites quickly. If some shortening results it is of no significance. If some angular deformity persists it is usually concealed by muscle covering. If angular deformity persists it is concealed in the flexed position of the elbow and becomes revealed only when the elbow is fully extended (a position in which the elbow is rarely viewed in ordinary postures of the body). These are facts which must be remembered when any elaborate or operative method for treating this bone is under consideration.

Sling or Collar and Cuff

It is surprising how few people realise the fundamental difference in the mechanics of a sling and a ' collar and cuff.' Few realise that the two are diametrically opposite in their mechanical action on the humerus, shoulder, and shoulder girdle.

A sling elevates the point of the elbow and thus applies a vertical *compression* force in the length of the humerus and on the shoulder joint. It must not therefore be used when treating a fracture of the humerus because it will cause overriding and lateral angulation.

A collar and cuff allows the weight of the elbow to generate a traction force on the shoulder and it tends therefore to elongate the humerus.

When treating fractures of the humerus a collar and cuff must be used. When treating fractures of the clavicle and dislocation of the acromio-clavicular joint, where it is necessary to elevate the shoulder, a sling is required.

Oblique or Comminuted Fractures of the Humerus

These can be adequately treated by nothing more elaborate than a U-shaped plaster slab, and a collar and cuff applied to the wrist with the arm bandaged to the side of the body with circular turns of a flannel bandage (Fig. 74, A, B). This simple method tends to be despised by those who fear permanent stiffness of the shoulder; but in young adults serious shoulder stiffness is not a frequent complication. This method of fixing the arm to the side of the chest was widely

99

adopted in the Middle East Force in 1941 for gunshot fractures of the shaft of the humerus; for purposes of transport the whole arrangement was made even more compact by applying plaster of Paris over the flannel bandage. When first used in this way it was only intended as a first-aid measure, because the transport of wounded with the arm abducted in a plaster spica was found to be impossible,

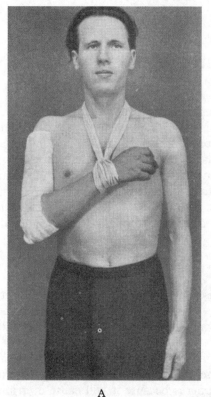 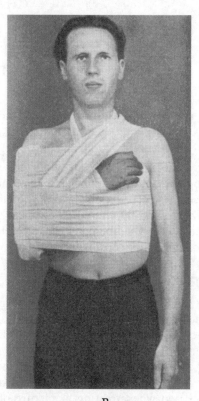

A B

FIG. 74

A, First stage of treatment of a fracture of the shaft of the humerus. The U-shaped slab is bandaged in position and collar and cuff applied.
B, Second stage. Encircling body bandage of domette applied.

but many surgeons continued to use it as a definitive method because the results were good and the method simple.

In contrast to this method, the more popular ' hanging cast ' method is open to serious mechanical criticism. In the first place the *hanging cast readily produces over-distraction of the humerus* (Fig. 75, A, B), though it would be more correct to say that it reveals the extensive tearing of soft parts which is impossible for distraction and for delayed union. In the second place the upper margin of the plaster, lying between the chest wall and the inner side of the arm, acts as a fulcrum and tends to induce lateral bowing at the fracture. *Lateral bowing can be prevented by bandaging the arm against the side of the chest*, a procedure which tends to cause medial bowing (Fig. 76, B). The hanging cast does not allow the shoulder joint to be exercised through any significant range, therefore exercise of the shoulder cannot be argued either in its support or against it.

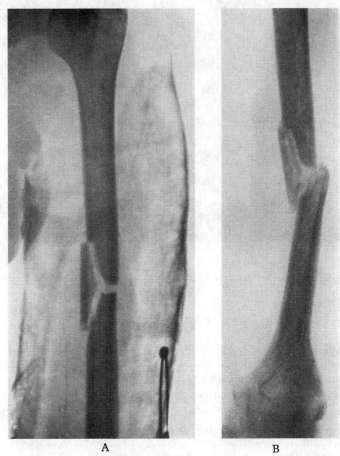

A   B

FIG. 75

A, Over-distraction of a fracture of the humerus produced by a hanging cast. This indicates extensive tearing of soft parts and delayed union can be predicted.

B, Result at four months showing complete absence of callus and late deformity.

Transverse or Blunt Oblique Fractures

These fractures of the humerus, unlike the oblique fractures, will usually require manipulative reduction; in doing this two details of technique are important, namely:

1. Synergic use of gravity, obtained by putting the patient in the sitting position.

2. Local anæsthesia, in order that the patient is able to sit.

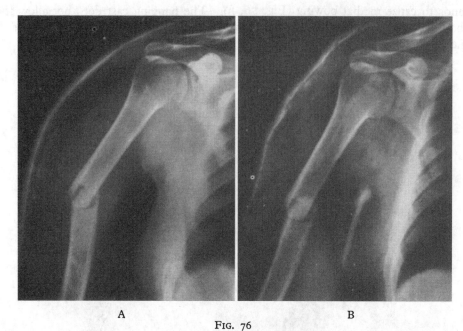

A   B

Fig. 76

Showing lateral bowing of a fracture of the mid-shaft of the humerus, and how bandaging arm firmly to the side improves position.

TECHNIQUE

A transverse fracture of the humerus is particularly suitable for reduction under local anæsthesia, provided that it is not more than two or three days old. The local anæsthetic is introduced into the fracture site (20 ml. of ½ per cent. Procaine) after entry into the hæmatoma has been checked by the re-aspiration of bloodstained anæsthetic back into the syringe. It is important to secure confidence by *giving this injection with the patient lying flat,* so that he has no inclination to faint; the subsequent painless manipulation, instead of being an ordeal, becomes a pleasant surprise when he sits up.

The patient is made to sit on a low stool, while an assistant steadies the shoulder by applying counter-extension with a looped towel passed under the patient's axilla; this towel may be conveniently hitched to a wall hook and the assistant thereby eliminated. An assistant now holds the patient's hand so that the forearm is horizontal and the surgeon applies a downward pull to the distal fragment by holding the epicondyles (Fig. 77). After moulding the fracture he tests whether the fracture is 'hitched' by its behaviour on applying an upward telescoping force on the lower fragment. If telescoping shows that overriding has not yet been overcome, the method of reduction by first increasing the angulation can be tried. The initial angulation in this fracture is concave posteriorly, owing to the superior tone of the triceps, and therefore the manipulation is to be based on the supposition that the soft-tissue 'hinge' lies on the dorsal aspect of the bone. All these manipulations should be done carefully to avoid damage to the musculo-spiral nerve.

If a reduction is obtained the surgeon maintains his hold of the epicondyles while an assistant applies a U-shaped plaster slab to the arm and a collar and cuff to the wrist; and the whole upper extremity is then bandaged to the side of the

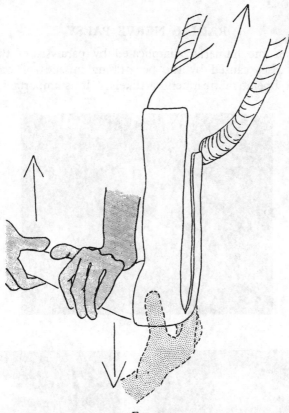

FIG. 77

Reducing a fracture of the humerus by downward traction and counter-traction against a loop of towel in the axilla. The circular wet gauze bandage is applied over the wet slab in this position and the limb adducted when the cast has set.

chest for four weeks (Fig. 74, B). It is important during the application of the U-shaped slab that the forearm should be held across the front of the chest, because the U-slab will not fit well if applied with the forearm externally rotated.

Post-operative

After four to six weeks the circular turns round the body are discarded and shoulder movement is started. A close-fitting U-slab is retained as a guard for the next two or three weeks.

103

Distraction

If a fracture of the shaft of the humerus shows distraction of the bone ends under the gentle traction of conservative methods it is evident that soft tissues have been seriously torn and delayed union can be suspected. It is therefore wise to proceed with a bone-graft without undue delay if the fracture is still freely mobile at eight or ten weeks.

RADIAL NERVE PALSY

In fractures of the humerus complicated by paralysis of the radial nerve, except in those cases caused by the penetrating missiles of warfare, complete recovery without operative treatment is likely. It is important, however, that

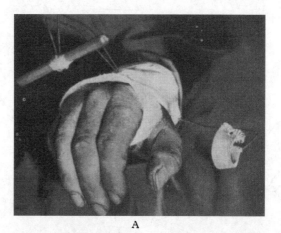

A

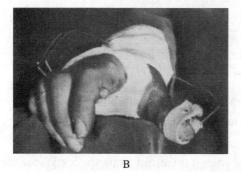

B

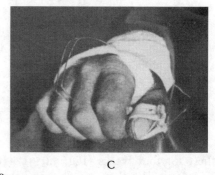

C

Fig. 78

'Lively' splinting (Capener) of fingers in radial palsy. This improvised method, using plaster and Kirschner wire, suffices until a detachable Brian Thomas splint can be obtained.

the fingers should be kept mobile during the period of recovery, and to do this some form of 'lively' splinting (Capener) is *essential*. A convenient method of applying this in default of specially constructed apparatus is illustrated (Fig. 78, A, B, C). The springs are made from Kirschner wires of appropriate thickness.

CHAPTER SEVEN

SUPRACONDYLAR FRACTURES OF THE HUMERUS IN CHILDREN

THE reduction of a supracondylar fracture of the humerus can become a comparatively simple feat if it is undertaken without delay and if the surgeon who has the first opportunity of treating it has a clear mental picture of its mechanism. The first reduction is the one most likely to succeed; after subsequent attempts the elbow becomes so indurated that the swelling may obstruct even the most expert manipulator.

ANATOMY OF THE FRACTURE

In the supracondylar fracture of the humerus the fracture line passes more or less transversely through the metaphysis at a variable distance from the epiphyseal line. When the fracture line is extremely close to the epiphyseal line it sometimes appears in the X-ray almost as an epiphyseal separation, but in every case a thin shell of the diaphysis is adherent to the distal fragment.

There are three elements in the displacement of the distal fragment of the supracondylar fracture: (1) posterior displacement, (2) lateral (or medial) displacement, and (3) rotary displacement.

In the manipulative reduction to be described, the rotary deformity will more or less correct itself under the influence of the tense fascial structures in the course of the preliminary phase of reduction by traction. An error of 10 degrees of rotation will not affect the functional or cosmetic result, though it will give rise to interesting appearances in the radiograph which need special comment (see below).

The two principal deformities, *i.e.*, the posterior and the lateral (or medial) displacement, are reduced in two quite separate stages:

Posterior Displacement

Posterior displacement of the distal fragment results from the distal end of the shaft of the humerus passing forwards into the antecubital fossa in front of the distal fragment. The intact soft structures, which form the 'tissue hinge' in this reduction, are the periosteum on the dorsal surface of the fracture and the tendon of the triceps which overlies it. The periosteal tube on the anterior aspect of the fracture is ruptured and the proximal end of the humerus passes through the rent to threaten the brachial artery or the median and radial nerves (Fig. 79, A, lateral view). This penetration of the humerus into the antecubital fossa results from the action of the superincumbent body weight as the child falls on the outstretched hand. The temporary incarceration of important structures, such as nerves or the brachial artery, between the two fragments is probably a common accompaniment of this displacement; but it will cause no permanent damage provided that the surgeon releases them **before flexing the elbow**. The incarcerated structures are released by the preliminary traction phase in reduction.

Lateral Displacement

Lateral displacement of the distal fragment can be either medial or lateral, being determined by the direction of the forces at the moment of the fall on the outstretched hand. The nature of this displacement is self-evident; but less obvious is the possibility that some varus or valgus displacement might persist after reduction which will be concealed by the flexed position of the elbow. Attempts to assess the presence of these angular deformities by direct X-ray of the fracture site are futile because a deviation of 10 degrees cannot be detected in the short distal fragment at such a proximity to the axis of angulation. The commonest residual deformity is a cubitus varus which, in a few cases, may necessitate osteotomy at a later date.

Soft Parts involved in the Reduction

The reduction of this fracture illustrates well the importance of a mental picture of the intact soft structures associated with broken bones, rather than allowing the X-ray shadows to dominate the mind (Fig. 79, A, B, C). The intact soft parts lie on the dorsal surface of the lower end of the humerus, the most important being the tendon of triceps and the dorsal periosteum. By keeping the triceps taut, at first by longitudinal traction in the axis of the *arm*, and later when the elbow is flexed as longitudinal traction in the axis of the *forearm*, the tendon of triceps will draw the distal fragment into the reduced position. When the elbow is fully flexed the moulding force of the triceps tendon is at its maximum.

Mechanical Analogy

A crude but valuable analogy which illustrates the mechanics of this reduction is offered in the application of a rubber tourniquet to a limb. The first movement in the application of a rubber tourniquet is the longitudinal stretching of the whole length of rubber in a straight line; the second movement is the winding of the rubber, while still stretched, round the fulcrum presented by the limb. In this sequence the direction of the traction changes continuously as the hand of the surgeon sweeps round the limb, though the longitudinal pull is maintained within the rubber (Fig. 80). In the mental picture for the reduction of a supra-condylar fracture the tendon of triceps is equivalent to the rubber of the tourniquet.

Thus far these remarks relate only to the mechanics of correcting posterior displacement of the distal fragment. The secret of correcting lateral displacement lies in the fact that **the elbow must never be flexed before lateral displacement**

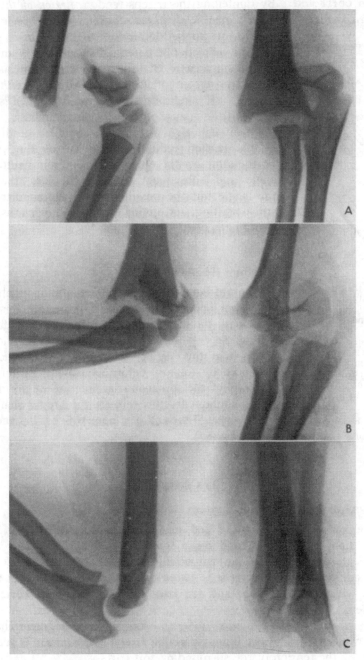

FIG. 79

A, Supracondylar fracture before reduction. Without knowledge of the
action of the soft parts the reduction of this fracture by closed manipulation might seem impossible !

B, Faulty reduction : lateral displacement had not been corrected by
adequate longitudinal traction, with the result that flexion locked the elbow
in the position of lateral displacement.

C, Complete reduction secured by remanipulation, this time extending
the elbow and applying traction prior to starting the flexion movement.

has been corrected. By tightening the triceps tendon, *flexion of the elbow will lock the fragments in whatever degree of lateral mal-alignment existed prior to flexion ; no pressure applied locally can then shift it.*

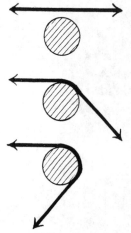

The correction of lateral displacement is an extremely simple manœuvre if adequate stress is laid on the initial movement of *longitudinal traction with the elbow straight.* If longitudinal traction is applied deliberately and with a pause for sufficient emphasis, the distal fragment will align itself with the shaft of the humerus by the tension induced in the surrounding soft parts. In the same act the elbow will acquire a neutral carrying angle and subsequent flexion will lock the elbow at this angle but the possibility of some angular deformity still persisting, and giving rise to cubitus varus, is always a lurking hazard.

FIG. 80

Indicating the mechanical analogy of the anchor tourniquet applied to a limb. The rubber is stretched before being wound round the limb. During the winding round the limb tension is maintained though the direction of traction is continually altering.

Rotatory Displacement

Not infrequently a post-reduction radiograph will show the lower end of the humerus projecting forwards as a spike with the distal fragment incompletely reduced below it (Fig. 81). J. K. Wright (personal communication) has shown that this ' spike ' is merely a radiological artefact produced by rotatory deformity. We often forget that at the level of the supracondylar fracture we are not dealing with an oblique fracture through the circular shaft of a bone but with a transverse fracture through the end of a bone which is flat and wide like the end of a paddle or spade (Fig. 82).

TECHNIQUE

Correction of Lateral Displacement

The elbow is gently extended and strong longitudinal traction is exerted by gripping the patient's wrist and distal forearm (Fig. 83). By this means the fragments are disengaged and any important structures incarcerated between them are released. In this manœuvre it is hoped that the distal end of the shaft of the humerus will retrace its path and fall back into the periosteal coverings from which it emerged anteriorly.

In the position of full extension under traction the distal fragment should move into line with the shaft of the humerus so that lateral displacement is automatically corrected by the tension of the surrounding soft parts.

It is important therefore to *pause at this stage to assess whether the lateral displacement has indeed been completely overcome before any attempt is made to hurry on to the next stage of the reduction.* If it has not been completely overcome,

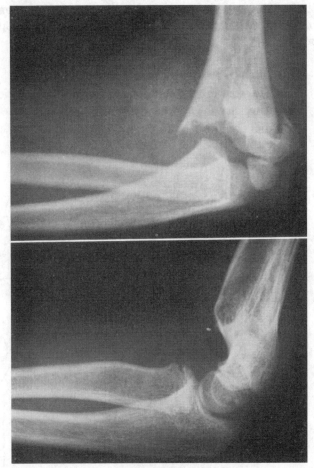

FIG. 81.—The forward pro-
jecting spike is the result
of misalignment in rotation.
Note how this deformity has
' remodelled ' two years sub-
sequently (lower figure).

FIG. 81

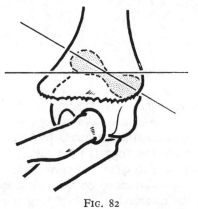

FIG. 82.—Rotatory deformity
(see text). Compare with
Fig. 81.

FIG. 82

some lateral pressure while the elbow is still extended may complete the reduction of the lateral displacement. In the extended position of the elbow the carrying angle will be obliterated and this will be the final appearance of the elbow when healed.

Correction of Posterior Displacement

The surgeon, still maintaining traction on the patient's hand with his ' active ' or ' reducing ' hand, grips the lower end of the humerus in his ' passive ' or ' fixing '

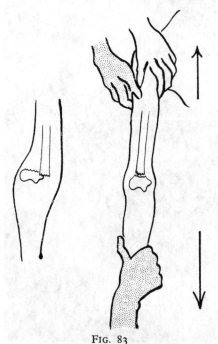

Fig. 83

Correction of lateral displacement by initial longitudinal traction. This alignment is produced by tension in the soft parts. This manœuvre releases any incarcerated artery or nerve which would suffer irreparable damage if the elbow were flexed without this having been done.

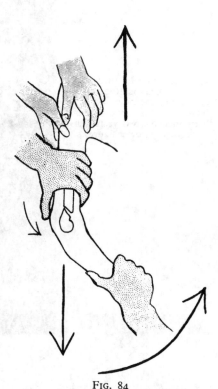

Fig. 84

Reduction started by flexing the elbow with traction still maintained.

hand to maintain counter-traction. The thumb of the fixing hand is applied over the olecranon.

With the active hand still applying longitudinal traction to the forearm, the active hand now flexes the elbow, *at the same time maintaining continuous traction in the axis of the forearm.* In order to maintain continuous traction a continuous counter-traction will have to be exerted by the fingers of the passive hand, and the direction of this counter-traction will have to change progressively as the elbow flexes (Fig. 84). *The critical point in the reduction occurs when the elbow is reaching the right angle ;* here the fingers of the passive hand are pulling the shaft of the humerus backwards while the pull of the active hand is directly drawing the distal fragment forwards (Fig. 85). The reduction is made or marred at this stage of the right-angle position of the elbow. Beyond the right-angle position further flexion does not improve the reduction but merely locks it by drawing the triceps tendon tight round the posterior surface of the fracture. If the reduction has not been secured at the right-angle position, further flexion will be resisted and may do damage if forced; **if lateral displacement has not been previously corrected, further flexion now will lock the elbow in lateral displacement.**

The reduction is now held by a collar and cuff in as much flexion as the

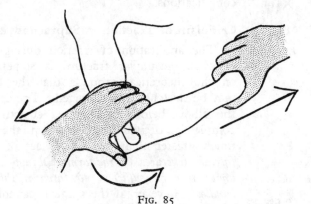

FIG. 85

Crucial phase of reduction; traction maintained but now 90 degrees away from the original direction. Distal fragment being pushed into place by pressure from the surgeon's thumb and tension in the triceps tendon.

presence of the radial pulse will tolerate and the elbow is kept inside the child's clothing.

It is unnecessary to apply plaster of Paris to this fracture. I have never seen a good reduction maintained in a plaster cast if the elbow is at a right angle.

Checking the Reduction Clinically

If the elbow is not grossly swollen, and particularly if the fracture is only a few hours old, the success of the reduction can usually be estimated by the ease with which flexion is attained. Even if considerable swelling is present, a sure method of estimating a successful reduction is to note the relation of the point of the elbow to the axis of the humerus. Even if there is considerable swelling *the ' point ' of the flexed elbow should lie in the axis of the humerus* and even slightly in front of it (Fig. 86). It is to be noted that by ' point ' of the elbow I mean the visible or palpable point discovered clinically; in these growing bones this does not necessarily coincide with the X-ray shadow, because growing cartilage is present. The degree of lateral displacement is often difficult to assess clinically if the elbow is swollen, but should be automatically corrected if longitudinal traction has been used as previously described.

If flexion of the elbow is secured easily, and if the point of the elbow lies correctly in the axis of the humerus or slightly in front of it, the surgeon should be able to say with some confidence that a reduction has been obtained, even before an X-ray is taken. Certainly this is true in a fresh initial reduction, but perhaps less so after previous unsuccessful manipulations have been attempted. Using the technique just described there should *never* be any necessity to perform open operations on these injuries except for nerve or arterial complications.

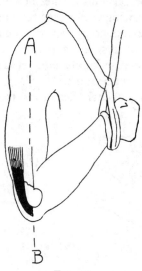

FIG. 86

Reduced fracture locked by the tension of the triceps tendon when the 90 degrees position of the elbow has been passed. This locking action is impossible at 90 degrees. The clinical test for reduction is seen by the point of the elbow lying in the axis of the humerus.

Criticism of Traction in Supracondylar Fractures

The application of traction during the reduction of a supracondylar fracture is sometimes criticised on the theoretical grounds that the brachial artery may be stretched and damaged. The danger of flexing the elbow before incarcerated structures have been completely drawn from between the fragments is much greater than the simple act of traction. *The fascial structures of the arm will not allow elongation under traction sufficient to threaten the neurovascular bundle.* However, if the surgeon cannot be convinced of the safety of applying traction with the elbow extended, it is still possible to apply longitudinal traction with the elbow at about 160 degrees instead of 180 degrees; but the patient's forearm must be grasped at its midpoint (*i.e.*, not holding the patient's hand) and this makes the subsequent movement of flexion combined with traction slightly difficult to execute precisely.

Difficulties with Circulation

The serious complication of Volkmann's ischæmic contracture is so well known that the importance of examining the radial pulse hardly needs much emphasis; but the absence of a radial pulse, on the other hand, is often possible without any fear of a Volkmann contracture. More important than the mere absence of radial pulse are: the warmth of the hand, the absence of extreme pain, the presence of circulation in the fingers, the absence of sensory loss, and the ability to extend the fingers passively.

In treating a child in whom there is a threat to the circulation the management of the case turns largely on the surgeon's concept of the cause of the obstruction. The obliteration of an artery by spasm is well known; but what factors cause this spasm, with the exception of local injury by the bone fragments, are less clearly understood. An important mechanical cause of arterial obstruction, which seems to me not to have received sufficient attention, results simply from flexing a tense and swollen elbow; it is possible that arterial spasm may later become superadded. These swollen elbows after a supracondylar fracture take on a turgidity akin to an inflated tyre, and it is the extended position of the elbow which reduces the internal pressure by allowing the greatest volume for its contents. Flexion of the unreduced elbow will increase the internal pressure. If a swollen elbow is flexed, a deep crease or kink will appear on the concave side which in itself is enough to obstruct the artery by direct pressure. This kink can be imitated by bending the finger of a rubber glove which has been distended with water (Fig. 87). If reduction is secured in a very swollen arm, it is often surprising how quickly the turgor of the tissues round the elbow will subside; after a successful reduction, often a distinct softening is appreciable by the time the child has recovered from the anæsthetic.

If, after preliminary traction in the manner described above, flexion of the elbow results in blanching of the hand and obliteration of the pulse when the 80 degrees position has been obtained (180 degrees equals extended position), the reduction will certainly slip if it is necessary to extend the elbow to 90 degrees. In such cases the child should be put to bed with skin traction applied from the elbow to the hand and with a plaster slab applied to hold the 90 degrees position. The arm should then be suspended from an overhead support with the child lying flat. If care is taken to see that the elbow cannot reach the surface of the bed, the weight of the arm will assist reduction and gravity will assist in the withdrawal of œdema. The suspension should be from a fixed point overhead, with an air space of about 2 inches between the bed and the elbow. After the first day and night a fretful child can usually be induced to put up with this situation, and it is not usually necessary to maintain it for more than four or five days (Fig. 88).

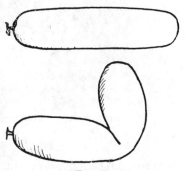

FIG. 87

Mechanical analogy of *kinking* a distended balloon to show the disastrous results of forcibly flexing the tensely swollen elbow of a supracondylar fracture.

In the illustration (Fig. 88) the limb is shown suspended with the elbow at about 100 degrees. This is because no plaster slab was used to hold the 90 degrees position achieved at manipulation. There is a danger that if the elbow is allowed to become partially extended, what was originally an incomplete, though satisfactory, reduction may relapse into considerable displacement. No plaster, by itself, will hold an incomplete reduction if the elbow is at 90 degrees, but when combined with traction it is possible to maintain whatever position was achieved by manipulation at 90 degrees. This is the only circumstance where I believe plaster is necessary in the supracondylar fracture.

In the arrangement of traction forces described by Dunlop (quoted and illustrated by Blount [1]) the counter-traction force is made more effective by passing a weighted strap over the front of the arm. This is a useful procedure

[1] BLOUNT, WALTER P. (1954). *Fractures in Children*, p. 35. Baltimore: Williams & Wilkins Co.

if, as the result of severe swelling, the elbow cannot be flexed as far as 90 degrees, but I find that it is rarely needed.

Remodelling of Displaced Supracondylar Fractures

It is well known that supracondylar fractures are capable of excellent remodelling and the recovery of full flexion which initially may be seriously blocked by the

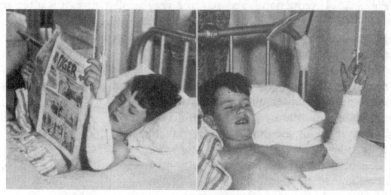

FIG. 88

Suspension of a swollen elbow when flexion to 90 degrees caused obliteration of pulse. (See text.)

forward projecting lower end of the upper fragment. This knowledge is very important in the handling of cases where several unsuccessful attempts to reduce

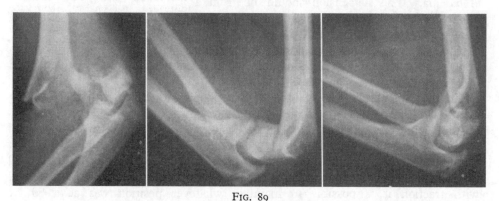

FIG. 89

Showing over-reduction of grossly displaced supracondylar fracture by too enthusiastic use of phase illustrated in Fig. 85. Over-correction reduced *secundum artem.*

have been made or where a threat to circulatory obstruction exists (Fig. 82, p. 109). So excellent can be the late results of remodelling that there is never any need to take any risk in re-manipulating this fracture. The only troublesome late deformity which persists after this fracture is cubitus varus.

Over-reduction of the Supracondylar Fracture

During the reduction of a supracondylar fracture care must be taken not to apply so much traction that the distal fragment is pulled completely in front of the lower end of the proximal fragment (Fig. 89); when the elbow is reaching the 90 degrees position the traction force in the axis of the forearm must therefore be intelligently moderated. The position of the point of the olecranon in relation to the axis of the humerus is just as useful in checking over-reduction as it is in checking failure to reduce.

CHAPTER EIGHT

FRACTURES OF THE RADIUS AND ULNA

IN this chapter we are only concerned with the treatment of fractures of the shafts of the radius and ulna in their middle thirds. There are many difficulties in treating the radius and ulna by closed manipulation ; closed methods can give excellent results, but the element of luck is rather prominent, and for this reason I am in favour of operative treatment. Some of the difficulties which damp enthusiasm for closed reduction are illustrated in the following sequence of catastrophes :

1. An excellent reduction may be secured by skilful manipulation.
2. The patient may suffer severe pain, with swollen fingers, because a close-fitting plaster is obviously necessary ; this causes the surgeon considerable anxiety, and may necessitate splitting of the plaster, thus causing further suffering to the patient unless a second anæsthetic is used.
3. When the swelling subsides there is a strong possibility of the initial reduction collapsing.
4. A second manipulation (sometimes the third anæsthetic) may therefore be necessary after fourteen to twenty-one days.
5. This may be followed by further pain and further swelling of the fingers.
6. An excellent reduction obtained initially is rarely ever retrieved by the second manipulation.
7. Delayed union of one or other bone may occur.
8. Limited pronation and supination may result after four to six months of plaster fixation.
9. External deformity may be so great as to be visible even to the patient.
10. Finally, bone grafting may be necessary in a forearm which is not fully mobile after six months of fixation. The operation may present considerable technical difficulty owing to mal-alignment of the fragments. The total disability following the grafting operation, after a further four months in plaster, will be about twelve months, the greater part of which time having been spent in plaster.

This unhappy sequence is certainly an extreme example of all the disasters which can follow the conservative treatment of this difficult fracture, but it illustrates the fact that by closed methods the results are not entirely under the surgeon's control. After operative treatment, on the other hand, there is practically no possibility of late deformity spoiling the result ; early movement is possible, and **if delayed union should result a bone graft can be substituted for the** plate with the minimum trouble and in a forearm already fully mobile at the time of grafting.

Against the operative treatment of forearm fractures in women, we must not ignore important cosmetic factors. A longitudinal scar on the radial aspect of the forearm is permanent and very disfiguring, because it always has a tendency to heal through a keloid phase. On the other hand, complete overriding of the forearm bones produces no external blemish if alignment is preserved. There is here scope for clinical judgment in which the patient's occupation will be considered. The case of a boy of eight years of age, illustrated in Fig. 90, gives food for thought ; this boy had a transverse fracture of the lower end of the radius with overriding of the fragments which defied two attempts to reduce by closed

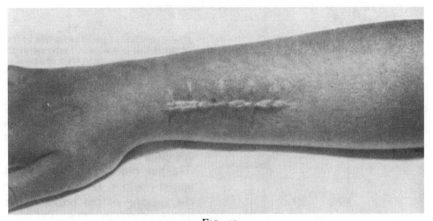

FIG. 90

Illustrating the cosmetic argument against the operative treatment of fractures of the forearm in young patients.

manipulation and eventually the ends were got into contact by directly exposing them. Had this small patient been a girl I would have advised strongly against operation because the overriding fracture would remodel completely in the course of three or four years. Blount [1] has published illustrations showing how completely the normal anatomy can be restored by remodelling in children's forearm fractures with overriding of the fragments.

The use of intramedullary nails in the forearm bones theoretically would avoid the unsightly scars inevitable if these fractures are plated. I have not been happy with my own attempts to insert intramedullary nails in the forearm, and for this reason I use plates whenever operative treatment is indicated.

TECHNIQUE OF CLOSED REDUCTION

Despite the disadvantages of the closed method it is important that the best method of performing it should be known, for there are many cases where operation is contraindicated.

[1] BLOUNT, WALTER P. (1954). *Fractures in Children*. Baltimore : Williams & Wilkins Co.

Disadvantages of Horizontal Technique

Perhaps the commonest method of attempting the closed reduction of this forearm fracture follows the technique described by Böhler in which traction is applied to the fingers, while counter-traction is applied at the elbow by a webbing sling attached to a hook on the wall.

The main objection to

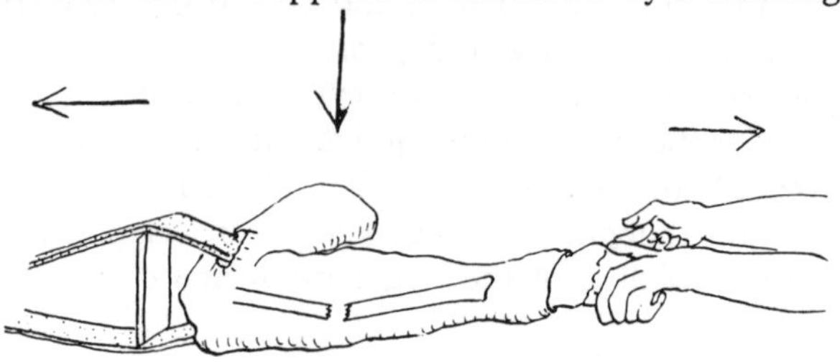

FIG. 91

Horizontal technique of reduction in fractures of the radius and ulna. The counter-traction sling prevents the application of a good plaster. Gravity tends to encourage sagging at the fracture site.

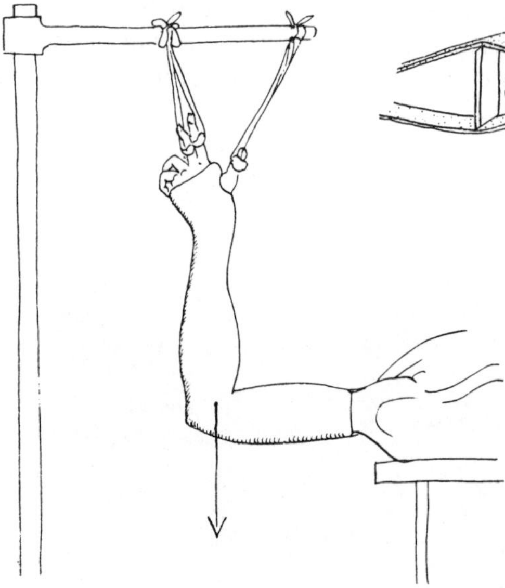

FIG. 92

Vertical position for reducing and plastering a fracture of the forearm. Counter-traction by gravity. Note position of digits to allow easy application of plaster through the first cleft. Gravity helps in alignment.

this method is that the counter-traction sling makes it impossible to apply a full-arm plaster except by applying it in two separate stages. Another objection is that the horizontal position favours deformity by the sagging of the bones under the action of gravity (Fig. 91).

By holding the forearm vertically, suspended from the thumb and index finger, the weight of the arm and proximal part of the forearm will apply its own traction and a full plaster can be applied in one stage.

In the vertical position of the forearm there is no tendency for the fragments to sag and parallel alignment is favoured (Fig. 92).

The Vertical Technique

The following technique includes several points which, though apparently trivial, contribute materially to ultimate success.

The patient is fully anæsthetised to secure relaxation. The forearm is suspended vertically by attaching 'monkey puzzles' or clove hitch knots to the thumb, index and middle fingers, and these are suspended from any convenient overhead frame (an intravenous drip-stand is very convenient because it allows the height to be varied). The thumb is suspended separately from the index and middle fingers to facilitate the passage of the plaster bandage round the palm (Fig. 92). The patient lies horizontally on the table and the height of the suspension is adjusted so that the arm is horizontal and, therefore, with the forearm vertical, the elbow is exactly at 90 degrees. A slight increase in traction to assist reduction can be applied by an assistant exerting downward pressure on the arm, or by gripping the epicondyles and pulling downwards.

The fracture is now manipulated by applied pressure at the level of the fracture, the surgeon squeezing the forearm between his hands with the ' squeezing ' grip shown in Fig. 93. During this procedure the forearm is best held in supination so that the squeeze separates the forearm bones from one another ; thereafter the forearm can be allowed to fall into the natural position of mid-pronation. An X-ray film should be taken at this stage to check the reduction.

If an X-ray shows that one or both of the bones are still overriding, it is obvious that the swelling of the forearm or the fibrous elements in the forearm are offering a mechanical barrier to elongation. It is useless in this case to repeat the same manipulation ; my own experience has been that the use of longitudinal traction continuously for several minutes, as recommended by Böhler, rarely succeeds, though when using local anæsthesia it might well be important. If, therefore, length is not secured in the first attempt, the second attempt should be made by the manœuvre of increasing the deformity followed by straightening the limb when apposition has been secured ; after this manipulation the forearm should again be suspended by the digits for the application of the plaster.

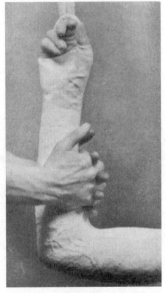

FIG. 93

The ' squeezing ' grip for reduction and for moulding the cast into an oval cross-section.

It is advisable to apply a single layer of wool before applying the plaster ; a skin-tight plaster provides no better mechanical fixation than a padded plaster skilfully applied, and the removal or splitting of a skin-tight plaster may necessitate an anæsthetic or otherwise inflict great discomfort on the patient.

The application of *adhesive felt pads to the head of the ulna, and particularly to the medial epicondyle at the elbow*, is a trivial detail but one strongly to be recommended ; these are often sources of great discomfort and may prevent the patient rehabilitating in the cast because of pain.

The plaster is applied from the knuckles to the lower part of the axilla with the forearm in mid-position. During the application of the plaster an assistant must hold the elbow by the epicondyles to prevent it swaying from side to side as the turns of the plaster are applied.

Two points in the application of this plaster deserve special emphasis :

1. THE THUMB

It is a common practice to cut away the plaster from the base of the thumb so as to expose the whole of the thenar eminence with the object of leaving the first metacarpal free to perform a complete circumduction at the carpo-metacarpal joint. This well-intended notion brings in its train an unfortunate sequel: the

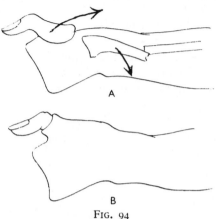

tendency for the radius to shorten by collapse of the distal fragment towards the ulna can logically be prevented only by some form of traction applied to the thumb; but cutting away the plaster from the thumb *invites* collapse of the radius by removing purchase on the thumb; the radius then collapses and the base of the thumb is drawn back against the margin of the plaster and a pressure sore develops at the base of the thumb (Fig. 94, A). To relieve this point of pressure futile attempts are often made to pack lint between the skin and the plaster; to cut the plaster farther back merely results in another pressure sore and further collapse of the radial fragment. For this reason I am convinced that **the thumb should always be enclosed up to the interphalangeal joint just as in the treatment of a scaphoid fracture.** This introduces a slight traction element to resist shortening and certainly makes the patient comfortable. If the thumb is brought round to oppose the fingers (as it should be in the treatment of a scaphoid fracture) there is no danger of stiffness even if the thumb is so fixed for twelve weeks (Fig. 95).

FIG. 94

A, If the thenar eminence is liberated from the plaster with the object of encouraging movement in the thumb, a pressure sore often results at the proximal part of the aperture. This is inevitable if the radius collapses towards the ulna.

B, By incorporating the whole thumb, as in the scaphoid plaster, a pressure sore at the base of the thumb is avoided.

2. THE OVAL CROSS-SECTION OF THE CAST

During the setting of the plaster it is important to apply the ' squeezing ' grip at the level of the fracture so as to mould the plaster into an oval cross-section (Fig. 93). This is a most important step; **if the cross-section of the plaster at the mid-forearm is circular the constricting action of the plaster tends to drive the forearm bones together; if the cross-section is oval this is avoided.** The padded plaster, compressed into an oval cross-section, can be regarded as exerting high pressure across the forearm in the narrow diameter, and low pressure in the long diameter (Fig. 96); the radius and ulna thus tend to float away from each other in the direction of low pressure. A more exaggerated exploitation of this principle was used by Böhler who incorporated two short lengths of wood in the plaster in an attempt to exert pressure between the fragments and open out the interosseous space; though experience has shown this to be a *dangerous* procedure I have no doubt that the principle is effective, for when pressure is applied by the finger tips between the bones of the forearm it is quite possible to feel the forearm bones separate from each other with a widening of the interosseous space.

GENERAL REMARKS

1. Patrick (1947) has shown *the danger of using a collar and cuff* to take the weight of the plaster ; he believes this to be the cause of the late angulation of

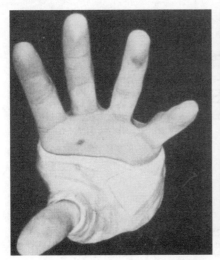
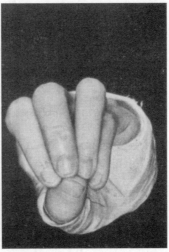

FIG. 95

Showing the ideal shape of the cast for function of the hand. Full opposition of the thumb is imperative.

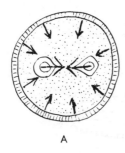
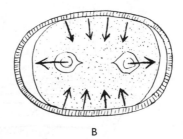

A   B

FIG. 96

A, A circular cross-section of the forearm part of the cast is to be condemned in a fracture of the forearm ; this encourages falling-in of the bones.

B, If the cast is compressed with an oval cross-section by the squeezing grip (Fig. 80) there is a tendency for the bones to float apart towards the zones of low pressure as the radial and ulnar borders of the cast.

both bones of the forearm, convex towards the ulnar border, which is such a common late development. This deformity results from the plaster maintaining a close grip on the distal half of the forearm, where the bones are practically subcutaneous, whereas the proximal half of the forearm is only loosely gripped by the plaster, being enclosed in large muscular bellies which rapidly shrink and waste. The dropping of the plaster at the elbow which is encouraged by the collar and cuff thus produces angulation. *If the elbow is supported by a sling and the*

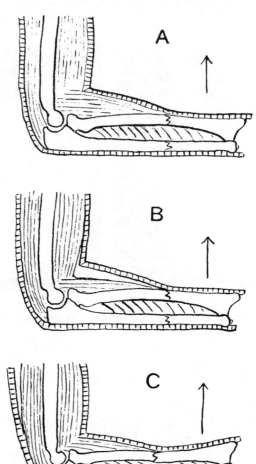

FIG. 97

Showing how a collar and cuff, applied to a forearm cast, can induce ulnar bowing (after Patrick). If held by a collar and cuff the plaster cast drops at the elbow when the forearm muscles waste; this produces ulnar bowing because the wrist is still held firmly by the cast. A sling is therefore to be preferred as it prevents dropping of the cast at the elbow.

plaster prevented from dropping at the elbow there is less tendency for this late deformity (Fig. 97).

2. The plaster should be retained continuously for twelve weeks before the

limb is examined for clinical union and therefore the plaster should be a good one from the start.

3. Should the plaster need changing for looseness or any other reason, the limb should be suspended by the digits to prevent angulation during this procedure.

4. Finger exercises are obviously of great importance, but of equal importance, though sometimes forgotten, is the need to maintain full movement in the shoulder; by insisting that the patient touches the back of the neck and the small of the back he secures full abduction, full internal rotation and full external rotation in two simple movements.

5. *Greenstick fractures of the forearm in children should never be treated in skin-tight plaster casts.* Because the greenstick fracture presents only an angular deformity it is ideally suited to fixation in a three-point splint. If the angular deformity is straightened, all that is needed is a padded plaster applied for three to four weeks and a perfect result will be obtained. It is horrifying to see the unnecessary suffering to these little patients which the application of a skin-tight plaster can often cause. Manipulation of a greenstick fracture often results in it becoming complete, and indeed it is advisable that the fracture should be deliberately completed to remove the ' spring action ' of the intact bridge which may induce the return of the original deformity (Fig. 51, p. 54). In a skin-tight plaster further swelling of the forearm will result in blue and swollen fingers. The subsequent splitting of the plaster may be so painful, unless an anæsthetic is given, that a permanent psychological resentment may develop against the idea of a hospital. Numerous cases of Volkmann's ischæmic contracture have been *caused by bad treatment* of this utterly trivial fracture.

6. The greenstick fracture of the forearm in children illustrates very clearly the dictum that to get a straight limb one must use a curved plaster (p. 51). The concavity of the plaster must be in the opposite sense from that of the original deformity which is usually concave dorsally (Fig. 98).

Late Angulation in Greenstick Fractures of the Radius

There are certain greenstick fractures of the radius which tend to develop a most disfiguring late deformity after an initially perfect reduction. Unless the surgeon knows this he will have the unpleasant experience of removing a plaster from a case which, till then, he has thought offered no difficulty, and finding to his chagrin the initial deformity of dorsal concavity of the radius (Fig. 99). Not only is this an ugly deformity, and one which causes the parents of the child great alarm, but if allowed to persist it may permanently limit pronation of the wrist. The fracture which is most susceptible to this late deformity is that involving the radius *when the ulna is intact*. Fractures of both the radius and the ulna seem to be less prone to this late deformity. The deformity is one of angulation, concave on the dorsal surface.

Whatever may be the actual mechanism of late dorsal angulation of the radius, one thing is certain, that *it defies all attempts at correction by the application of local force over the convexity*. Attempts to remanipulate the fracture while the callus is still soft appear to be frustrated by the presence of the intact ulna which shields the fracture from the full effect of any local corrective force.

If the callus is still soft the deformity can be corrected easily by forcible pronation of the distal fragment. The reason for this is that the proximal fragment reaches the end of its range of pronation while the distal fragment is still in some supination as a result of the angular deformity. By forcing the wrist into full pronation the proximal fragment reaches full pronation before the distal and cannot pronate any farther, so the soft callus at the fracture

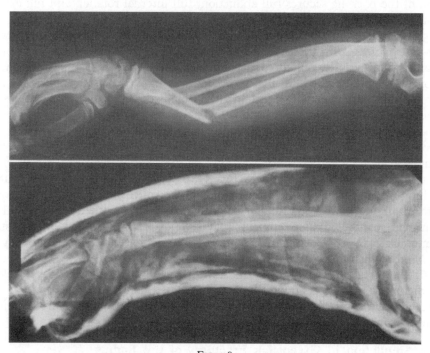

FIG. 98

Three-point plaster in action. A straight limb is produced by a curved plaster. Compare Fig. 48, A, page 51. Curvature of plaster is opposite to original deformity.

line must yield and allow the distal fragment to align itself with the proximal (Fig. 100). To hold this reduction it is necessary to apply the plaster with the wrist in practically full pronation; to hold the pronated position, it will be necessary to incorporate the elbow.

A similar mechanism occurs in the treatment of the Colles' fracture in the adult (p. 131). In the Colles' fracture the deformity of 'dorsal tilt' is prevented by locking the wrist in strong pronation.

Delayed Correction of Deformities in Children

The unsuspected recurrence of angular deformity in greenstick fractures of the forearm, while concealed in plaster, is an annoying event if it takes the

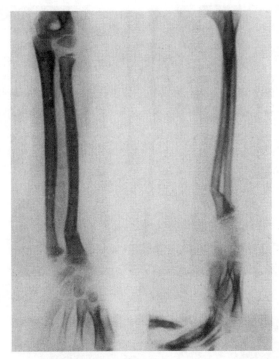

FIG. 99

Late dorsal tilt of greenstick fracture of radius occurring spontaneously inside the plaster. This can be prevented only by fixing in pronation, and is especially important if the ulna is intact.

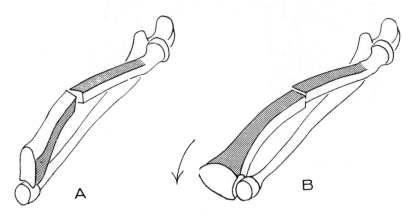

FIG. 100

Illustrating how a deformity of the radius which appears to be one of angulation, concave dorsally, in the presence of an intact ulna, has in fact an important element of supination in the distal fragment.

125

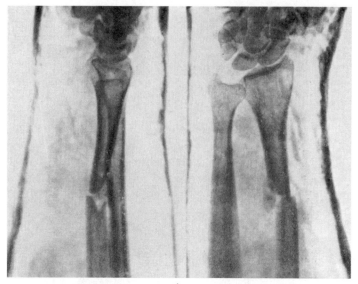

A

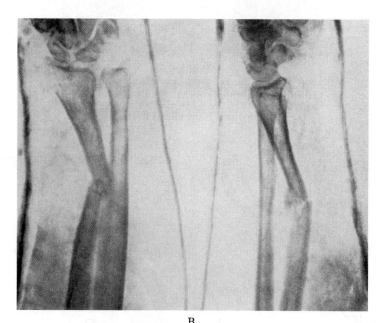

B

FIG. 101

A, Fracture through middle and lower thirds of the radius in good
positions in plaster.

B, Typical late collapse of the reduced position. This type of case
should always be treated by internal fixation.

surgeon by surprise and is not discovered until the plaster is removed. Parents, quite understandably, may be more annoyed about this happening to their children than if it had happened to themselves, and do not easily forgive the surgeon. This complication is very prone to happen if a greenstick fracture is not ' completed ' during manipulation, and is due to the elasticity of the bone or the tension of intact fascial structures on the concave side of the deformity.

However, if the surgeon specifically looks for the recurrence of the initial deformity at an early stage (*i.e.*, at four weeks) by taking an X-ray through the plaster, it can very easily be corrected while the callus is soft. When the fracture is ensheathed in callus the fragments can be moulded precisely into the desired position without fear of further recurrence. There is much to be said in favour of this as a planned ' two-stage ' procedure, especially if the original fracture is very mobile, and it is wise to mention it to the parents immediately after the first reduction ; if late ' moulding ' is not needed no harm is done, but if later it is needed the parents know the surgeon has the matter under control.

Fractures of the Lower Third of the Radius

A common fracture of the adult radius occurs at the junction of its lower and middle thirds, without fracture of the ulna ; the radius collapses towards the ulna and results in subluxation of the lower radio-ulnar joint (Fig. 101, A, B). The deformity in this fracture is particularly prone to recurrence even if manipulative reduction has been complete, but **if manipulative reduction has been only partially successful one can guarantee with absolute certainty that complete relapse of the initial deformity will take place in the plaster.** In this fracture operative treatment with internal metallic fixation is *always* advisable except in the aged.

CHAPTER NINE

THE COLLES' FRACTURE

I T is a fortunate thing that excellent functional results usually follow the common Colles' fracture, because disappointing anatomical results occasionally develop even in the most skilful hands. Though in general it is fair to class this injury as a minor fracture, this is not always the case, because the group includes a substantial number of comminuted fractures which would demand elaborate mechanical treatment if perfect anatomical restoration were to be the most important aspect of the problem.

From the student's point of view it is confusing that this common fracture is satisfactorily treated by a method which transgresses two of the basic principles of fracture treatment because, as will be shown later, the dorsal plaster slab is mechanically unsound as a method of fixation, and the position of flexion of the wrist is contrary to the general rule of splintage in the optimal position for function. Here, however, is an example of a method which is sanctioned by results and by convenience rather than theory, and these are very important practical matters in a busy clinic.

ANATOMY OF THE FRACTURE

The triple displacement of a Colles' fracture, *i.e.*, dorsal shift, dorsal tilt, and radial shift of the distal fragment, constitutes the classical 'dinner-fork' deformity known to every student. Less obvious, but more important as regards treatment, are the ruptured soft parts which accompany this displacement. The tissue which is ruptured on the volar aspect of the fracture is the periosteum, while on the dorsal surface of the fracture the periosteum and the fibrous part of the tendon sheaths remain intact and thus constitute the soft tissue 'hinge' which is the key to reduction of the displacement (Fig. 102).

In elderly patients the Colles' fracture is always comminuted, and this is responsible for the slipping of the reduction which is a rather common late feature in this injury. Comminution of the dorsal cortex invites backward tilting of the distal fragment because *it removes the strut which would otherwise be provided by the accurate reduction of an intact dorsal cortex.* When the fracture is impacted the shaft of the radius, which constitutes the proximal fragment, becomes deeply embedded in the cancellous bone of the distal fragment, and when it is disimpacted the cavity left in the distal fragment fills with nothing more substantial than blood clot (Fig. 103).

It will be seen therefore that many Colles' fractures possess little or no stability following reduction and *in theory* the tendency to collapse in this type

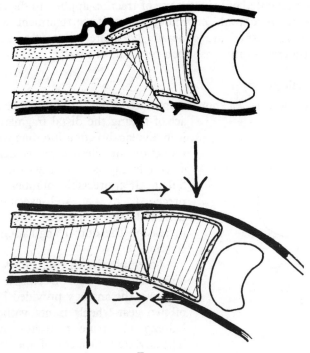

FIG. 102

Showing the soft parts involved in a Colles' fracture. The soft-tissue hinge lies on the dorsal aspect, and it is this which must be maintained under tension to produce, and to hold, the reduction.

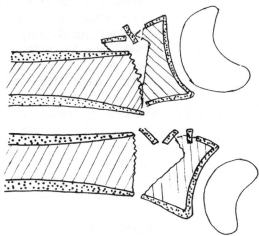

FIG. 103

Showing the cause of late collapse in the comminuted Colles' fractures so often encountered in the aged. The comminution of the dorsal cortex removes the solid strut which normally prevents redisplacement, and the cavity in the cancellous bone contains nothing more substantial than blood clot.

129

of case could be prevented only by the use of traction applied to the distal fragment. Traction in this fracture would enormously complicate treatment and, because the results of a simple method are generally adequate, matters of convenience are more to be considered in this case than mechanical ideals.

Mechanical Analogy

Many stable fractures, *i.e.*, non-comminuted cases, can be reduced by the simple act of flexing the distal fragment and pressing it in a volar direction into line with the radius ; reduction in these cases is demonstrated by a convincing snap. But this method will fail in an appreciable number of cases unless preceded by a well-executed movement designed to disimpact the fragments by increasing the dorsal angulation and applying traction.

To emphasise the *importance of preliminary disimpaction* in the treatment of a Colles' fracture, the analogy provided by the meshing of two gear-wheels is not without interest in helping to create a useful mental picture. The serrated surfaces of the fracture can be regarded as the teeth of two gear-wheels which have been erroneously meshed. Let us regard the distal wheel as being erroneously meshed by a backward rotation of two teeth in relation to the proximal. Simple pressure cannot restore the correct relation of the two wheels without shearing the teeth, and simple forward rotation will still leave the distal wheel out of alignment by the distance of two teeth (Fig. 104). It is obvious that the distal wheel will have to be separated by traction to disengage the teeth and then **by increasing the backward rotation** the 'dorsal teeth' can be correctly enmeshed ; forward rotation of the distal wheel will now result in correct alignment (*i.e.*, the 'volar teeth' will now come into alignment when flexion is complete).

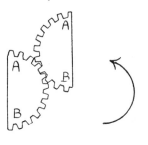

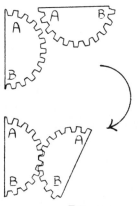

FIG. 104

Mechanical analogy in reducing a Colles' fracture.

A, Fracture in displaced position (teeth incorrectly meshed).

B, Fracture distracted and backward angulation increased in order to mesh the dorsal teeth correctly.

C, Flexion will now bring the volar cortices correctly into register.

TECHNIQUE

It is important to have full muscular relaxation by general anæsthesia ; 'smash and grab' under N_2O is useless.

In the reduction of a **left** Colles' fracture the surgeon grips the patient's forearm with his left hand sited on the volar aspect so that his thenar eminence is under the proximal fragment. The right hand of the surgeon is then applied to the distal fragment, the thenar eminence being sited on its dorsal surface.

Throughout the subsequent three movements which produce the reduction it will be observed that **the left hand of the surgeon remains stationary, acting as the passive hand or 'vice,' while the active part of the manipulation is executed by the right hand alone.**

Step 1. Disimpaction

An assistant takes hold of the elbow and offers counter-traction. The surgeon applies traction with the right hand, sited as just described, at the same time

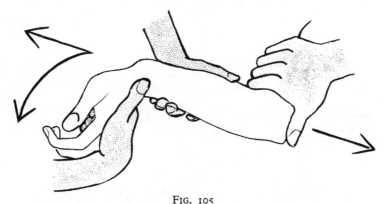

FIG. 105

Disimpaction and increasing the backward angulation.   Traction maintained.

increasing the deformity by dorsiflexing the distal fragment ('re-engaging the dorsal teeth,' Fig. 105).

Step 2. Reduction

With traction still maintained, by means of the right hand the surgeon presses the distal fragment in a volar direction and then follows this with the final flexion of the wrist. The thenar eminence of the left hand applies counter-pressure against the proximal fragment during this movement (Fig. 106). *At the end of this movement the fracture is fully reduced, but it would slip if the traction force were released or if one of the two forces applying pressure and counter-pressure were removed.*

Step 3. Locking the Fracture by Pronation

The fracture is now rendered stable by the surgeon pronating his right hand, thus carrying the distal fragment into pronation and *at the same time deviating the patient's wrist towards the ulna* (Fig. 107). **If pronation is maintained the reduction will hold without traction.** This is explained by the fact that the proximal fragment in a Colles' fracture can only slip out of alignment with the distal fragment by moving in the direction of pronation, but, if the forearm is

131

already in full pronation, it cannot therefore move any farther in order to lose alignment with the distal fragment.

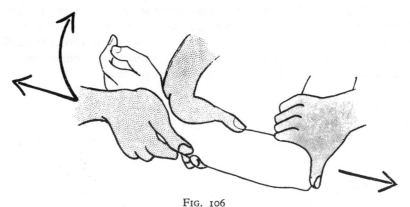

FIG. 106

Robert Jones grip applied. Pressure is applied with 'reducing' hand on distal fragment against the counter-pressure on the proximal fragment from the 'anvil' hand. Traction maintained.

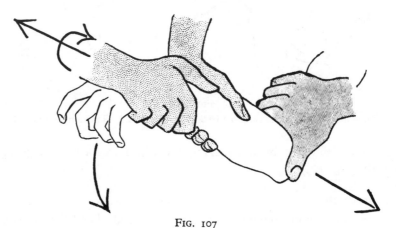

FIG. 107

Locking the reduction by pronation. The 'anvil' hand remains stationary while the pronation is done entirely by the 'reducing' hand. The wrist is forced into ulnar deviation by this same manœuvre.

Application of the Plaster

The application of plaster to a Colles' fracture is a tricky business which is personal to many surgeons and rather defies description. Faulty reductions are more often the result of clumsy plaster technique than faulty manipulation. I have found the following procedure convenient for both the surgeon and the assistant.

A quick-setting plaster slab is laid on the back of the forearm and bandaged in position with a wet gauze bandage. To facilitate the unobstructed work of the assistant who is applying the plaster the surgeon adopts the hold illustrated (Fig. 108), in which the thumb is taken in one hand and the fingers in the other ;

no traction is used and the stability of the reduction depends on maintaining strong pronation. In this position ulnar deviation and slight palmar flexion is possible. To reach this holding-grip it is necessary for the surgeon to slide his hand from the position in Fig. 107 to that in Fig. 108 with some care, but if strong pronation is maintained the fracture will not slip. The only difficulty in the application of the slab in this position is that the wrist is sometimes almost upside down during the application of the plaster slab and the dorsal surface of the wrist is facing the floor.

When the plaster has been completed the surgeon resumes his hold in Step 3

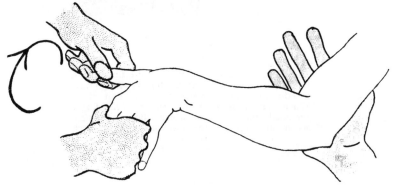

FIG. 108

Plastering position. Held in strong pronation the traction can be released without danger of the fracture slipping. Note ulnar deviation, separation of the thumb to facilitate passage of the bandage and exclusion of the fifth finger from the grip. Sometimes the pronation needed makes application of the plaster slab a little awkward as the wrist is almost upside down.

(Fig. 107) and moulds the plaster at the points of local pressure on the two fragments (see below) until the slab has hardened.

Note in Fig. 108 that the fifth finger is excluded from the grip of the surgeon's hand; this is explained in Fig. 109 as a means of preserving the normal width of the palmar arch in the completed plaster.

The Plaster Slab

For mechanical reasons the *ideal* plaster splint for this fracture would be a complete circular cast; but in Britain this is not often used because a plaster slab is more convenient in this very common fracture and the results of this method are quite adequate. The ideal cast would be moulded into a three-point system against the volar aspect of the proximal fragment and the dorsal aspect of the distal fragment (Fig. 110). To deter the fracture from slipping into radial displacement (*i.e.*, shortening of the radius) the ideal cast would have the thumb incorporated as far as the interphalangeal joint as in the case of a scaphoid plaster. From time to time various workers have suggested that the forearm should be held in full pronation by incorporating the elbow in the plaster, but this is unnecessary and delays rehabilitation. Permanent pronation of the forearm

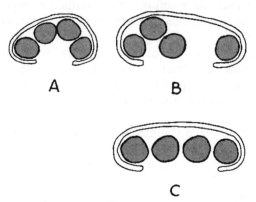

FIG. 109

Showing reason for excluding the fifth finger from
the grip in Fig. 108. If all fingers are gripped
together the plaster which results is that of A.
When plaster is applied with the fifth finger
excluded, this gives B, which allows of ample
accommodation for the transverse palmar arch
as at C.

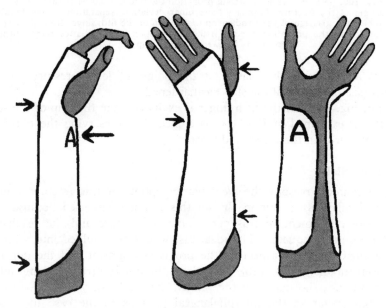

FIG. 110

The radial plaster slab. Slight palmar flexion. Considerable ulnar deviation.
Thick plaster at the point marked A in order to make the plaster conform to
the principles of a three-point splint.

is unnecessary if the fragments are held in alignment by the local moulding of the plaster on the volar and dorsal aspects as part of a three-point system.

Despite the theoretical superiority of the complete cast, the plaster slab scores heavily as regards convenience; but to use a slab effectively there is one matter of such importance that it cannot be too much emphasised. **The plaster slab should never be merely a dorsal slab, it must always be a radial slab;** to emphasise the importance of this I would suggest that in the treatment of the Colles' fracture the use of the term dorsal slab should be abolished and the name radial slab insisted upon. For a slab to exert a three-point action it is essential that the slab should reach the midline of the forearm on the volar aspect (Fig. 110). **On the volar aspect it should be thick enough to take a permanent impression from the surgeon's thenar eminence** while the plaster is setting. It is a common error to find a dorsal slab applied with the edges so thin at the point where they overlap on to the volar aspect of the wrist that no three-point action could possibly be maintained. Many good reductions are allowed to slip by the slab being a dorsal strip confined to the flat surface of the back of the wrist, thus making it impossible to use a three-point system. By the same token the reappearance of radial shift after successful reduction is usually due to the use of a flat slab confined to the dorsum of the forearm; **only by having a deeply curved splint applied to the radial aspect of the wrist is there any chance of preventing late radial deviation.**

Assessing the Reduction by X-ray

It is sometimes embarrassing to find in the end result a noticeable radial displacement of the hand which had not been previously suspected. Late radial deviation in a Colles' fracture is the only deformity which need present any serious problem; it must therefore be kept in the forefront throughout treatment. It will usually be found that careful observation of the levels of the radial and ulnar styloids will be a fairly useful guide to the presence of radial slip, but some cases will be found where quite a shapely wrist results even when the styloids are at equal levels. A useful guide to the possibility of radial deviation is in the shape of the plaster as seen in the X-ray; the shadow of the cast should always show as a straight line on the radial side but should have a concavity on the ulnar border (Fig. 111, c).

RESECTION OF THE LOWER END OF THE ULNA

When an ugly external deformity is encountered in a mal-united Colles' fracture it can be easily corrected by Darrach's operation (Fig. 112). This simple but most effective operation concerns the resection of the head of the ulna together with about 1 inch of the adjacent shaft. By this single procedure (1) the prominence of the ulnar styloid is removed, (2) the pain arising in the subluxated distal radio-ulnar joint is abolished, and (3) rotary movement at the wrist is restored to normal. The operation entails only three weeks of post-operative disability and the benefits which accrue will reveal themselves within six weeks. **With**

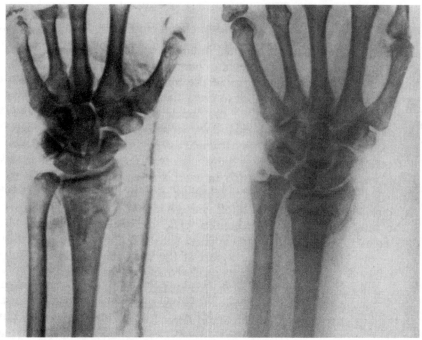

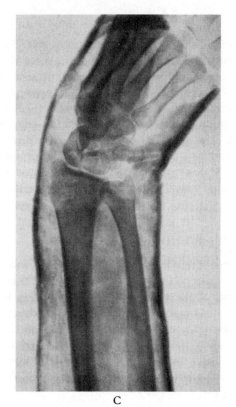

Fig. 111

A, Showing a fair reduction of a comminuted fracture but a bad plaster in neutral position.

B, Showing the inevitable late result of radial deviation.

C, X-ray appearance of a Colles' plaster in strong ulnar deviation.

the certain knowledge that a gratifying result can be obtained after this operation, it is wiser to accept a radial deviation in a mal-united Colles' fracture rather than to attempt remanipulation. In young patients the slipping of a Colles' fracture usually results from inexpert treatment, but the slipping of a Colles' fracture in elderly patients is to be regarded almost as a natural sequel, and attempts to remanipulate are likely to fail because further absorption of comminuted bone fragments is likely to occur. Having accepted a radial

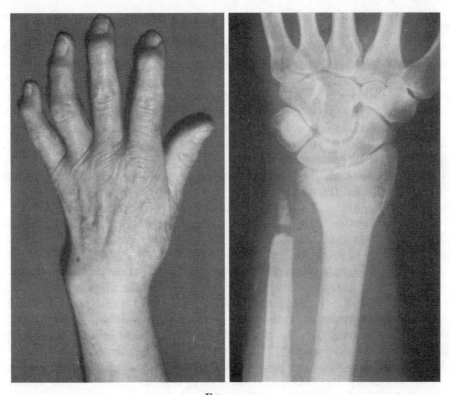

FIG. 112

Ugly deformity of radial deviation cosmetically corrected by resection of lower end of the ulna. This also restores full rotation and abolishes residual pain round the prominent head of the ulna.

deviation in an elderly patient, the splint should not be retained too long ; fixation should be abolished after three weeks, and mobilisation of the wrist should then be started. Resection of the ulnar styloid can be performed two or three months later if the patient is dissatisfied with the appearance or has persistent pain over the ulnar styloid.

The very best results of resection of the lower end of the ulna are in cases where there has been a serious block to pronation and supination. Not many patients will accept the idea of resection of the ulna if movement is reasonably good, and it is very important to realise that what causes most dissatisfaction with patients after a Colles' fracture is *pain* round the excessively prominent head of the ulna. They are not usually much bothered by slight deformity. It is important to realise that this pain will disappear spontaneously though it may last as long as one year. If they are firmly reassured about this the vast majority will be quite content.

FUTURE DEVELOPMENTS IN THE TREATMENT OF THE COLLES' FRACTURE

It has to be confessed that the conservative treatment of the Colles' fracture often leaves something to be desired in the cosmetic result, though rarely in the functional result. This is particularly so when the results of work done by young residents is considered, though even experienced operators occasionally have disappointing cosmetic results from the Colles' fracture. The perfectionist will continue to look for a method offering greater precision than the conservative method in order to eliminate the tendency to late displacement, and it is therefore the purpose of this section to examine how far mechanical elaboration of the treatment of the Colles' fracture is justifiable and in what directions future research might profitably be encouraged.

Numerous attempts have been made in the past to improve the anatomical results of the Colles' fracture by holding the wrist in full pronation throughout the early phase of splintage. This has been done by incorporating the elbow in the fully pronated plaster. This technique, though anatomically sound, is physiologically bad, because the elderly patients fail to recover supination if fixed in an extreme position of pronation for several weeks.

The Colles' fracture shortens the radius and tends therefore to subluxate the lower radio-ulnar joint, so damaging the triangular fibrocartilage at its attachment to the ulnar styloid. To hold the radial styloid down to its normal level it is obvious that, theoretically, some form of traction is needed. External skeletal fixation has been tried (*i.e.*, the Stader splint) and workers in Toronto have been enthusiastic about this method. Similar claims for comfort and for precision of holding of the reduction have been made for internal fixation using the Rush nail.

The fundamental criticism of maintaining the full length of the radius by mechanical methods is based on the biological principles of osseous union and joint movement outlined in Chapter I. The Colles' fracture is a fracture of cancellous bone, and four to six weeks after such a fracture I believe that union will be present only at the points where the cancellous fragments are in direct contact. If the radius is pulled out to its full length a cavity will be made inside the fracture which will not fill with new bone until many weeks have elapsed; it will fill only by the slow spread of osteogenesis from the points of initial contact and not by callus being 'thrown out' to fill the cavity. If the radius is pulled out to full length, initial union will be by a fragile bridge on the volar aspect with defective consolidation on the dorsal aspect and with a central cavity filled with fibrous tissue. If the apparatus maintaining length is removed after four weeks, there will be a tendency to collapse, and even if gross collapse does not occur, I believe that the threat will be manifest in a stationary, or even retrograde, phase in rehabilitation. *If consolidation is unsound the power of grip and the function of the wrist will be inhibited until sound osseous consolidation has been achieved.* It is during the phase of inhibited function which accompanies unsound consolidation that permanent joint stiffness develops. The Colles' fracture is therefore an excellent instance of what I believe is an axiom in the treatment of any fracture, namely, that the best way to functional recovery is by striving primarily for sound osseous union, and any factor in treatment which might delay osseous consolidation carries with it the danger of some permanent impairment of joint function.

On these biological grounds the fundamental approach to the treatment of the Colles' fracture must be to permit some collapse of the cancellous bone so as to achieve contact over a large area. The key to conservative treatment is therefore ' controlled collapse,' and provided that steps are taken to concentrate on preventing gross radial displacement the cosmetic appearance of the wrist will be acceptable. Under this regime the power of the grip will rapidly return and this in its turn may exert some beneficial compression stimulus on the cancellous bone of the fracture.

A Clinical Experiment

If traction is likely to delay consolidation by holding open a cavity in the lower end of the radius, it would seem logical to hold the radial styloid at its normal level by packing bone chips into the cavity left after reduction, and in this way the patient would theoretically compress the bone chips at each attempted movement of gripping. Claims for good results by this technique in the treatment of depressed fractures of the tibial plateau and in depressed fractures of the os calcis have been made by various workers in the past. To test this theory six Colles' fractures were operated in this way, using refrigerated bank bone.

The fracture line was exposed through a small incision at the base of the radial styloid, and while the fracture was held in the position of reduction by the assistant applying traction to the thumb, chips of bone were packed into the cavity to strut the fracture apart. In several cases a whole segment of rib was driven in as a wedge. Inspection of the size of the cavity in the distal fragment was an impressive confirmation of the instability of a Colles' fracture in the reduced position. At the conclusion of the operation the stability against shortening was gratifying, but during convalescence several of them collapsed in spite of the inserted bone (Fig. 113); this suggests that the dead bone of the graft did not take part in rapid union and was still exerting a delaying action on consolidation. However, an outstanding feature of the post-operative recovery was the absence of swelling and pain in the fingers which is such a common sequel to the Colles' fracture treated in plaster. This circulatory embarrassment is due to collapse of the fracture, rendering the wrist shorter and wider than it was at the moment when the plaster was applied with the fracture fully reduced. With this experimental operative technique a *padded* plaster could be used, because early collapse was prevented and no constriction developed. Despite this attractive and most important feature, it was felt that the operative method was unsuitable for routine use in a busy hospital and that in the hands of those on whom the reduction of

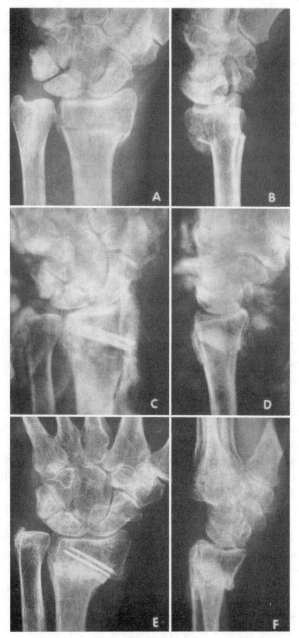

FIG. 113
See text.

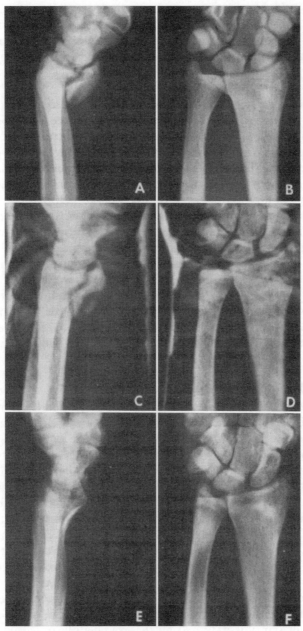

FIG. 114

Reversed Colles' fracture (Smith's fracture). Reduced, and held
in plaster, in supination. The simple 'cock-up' position,
logically the reverse of that used for the Colles' fracture, will
not hold this reduction.

most of these fractures devolve in British hospitals there would be complications making it unjustifiable; but the technique may well be of occasional use in selected cases and in expert hands. It is a matter of opinion whether perfect anatomical restoration with a surgical scar on the exposed radial aspect of the wrist is cosmetically superior to slight radial deviation without a surgical scar.

Delayed Reduction of the Colles' Fracture

The Colles' fracture is eminently suitable for delayed reduction and indeed I believe that whenever possible the method of choice is to permit the main swelling of the wrist to occur before attempting reduction. If the fracture is reduced and plastered immediately, or within an hour or two of having been sustained, severe swelling of the fingers is almost certain to occur, causing great pain and the necessity for splitting the plaster (and the splitting of the plaster can be a very painful procedure even if only a plaster slab has been used). Severe swelling of the fingers is all too common after a Colles' fracture and is a threat to ultimate function. A little common sense and clinical judgment must be used in recommending delayed reduction, and obviously some patients will be having pain as a result of the deformity and pressure on neurovascular structures, and delayed reduction should only be considered in patients who have little or no spontaneous resting pain. If suitable for delayed reduction a light padded cast can be applied to the recent Colles' fracture and the patient brought back at a more convenient time twenty-four to forty-eight hours later, by which time the patient will be fully prepared for anæsthesia, and much less finger swelling will be encountered after reduction.

Reversed Colles' Fracture (Smith's Fracture)

The reversed Colles' fracture, and the anterior marginal fracture of the radius, is a fracture-dislocation of the wrist in which the carpus is subluxated in a palmar direction. Though the displacement is easy to reduce by applying traction there is always a strong tendency for redisplacement in plaster when traction is removed. It is traditional to recommend that the wrist should be splinted in dorsiflexion, because the deformity is the reverse of a Colles' fracture, and pious hope is expressed in the advice of those who recommend that the shattered anterior lip of the radio-carpal joint can be moulded back into position by local pressure at the time of the reduction. It has been pointed out to me by F. Brian Thomas of Hereford that the reversed Colles' fracture can often be held in the reduced position by applying a plaster with the wrist in *full supination*. It is necessary to incorporate the elbow in plaster in order to hold the fully supinated position. In full supination the tendency for the radius to fall into pronation automatically forces the fragments into the reduced position. That this very simple technique may be the answer to this very difficult injury is indicated by the example illustrated in Fig. 114.

My objection to the treatment of the Colles' fracture in full pronation, by incorporation of the elbow in the plaster, does not apply here because the displacement of the Smith's fracture is so much more disabling than Colles' and often occurs in younger patients.

CHAPTER TEN

THE BENNETT'S FRACTURE

OPINIONS vary considerably on the frequency of late symptoms following unsatisfactory reductions of a Bennett's fracture. Casualty officers do not usually find it an easy fracture to reduce, and because it is also quite a common injury, one can presume that numerous cases must be treated inexpertly every year ; but even so, the number of cases presenting themselves with symptoms of traumatic arthritis is remarkably few. However, this is no reason why a high standard of manipulative reduction should not be expected. The reduction of this fracture presents no great mechanical difficulty but it demands from the surgeon a fine sense of touch, and for this reason the injury could well be used as a ' passing-out ' test for the student of closed reduction.

ANATOMY OF THE FRACTURE

As its alternative name implies, the ' stave ' fracture is often sustained in a bout of fisticuffs. An ill-delivered blow transmits force in the line of the thumb while in flexion, thereby shearing off the anterior part of the base of the metacarpal, and so allowing the bone to escape from the joint in a dorsal direction. The volar ligament of the carpo-metacarpal joint remains intact and this is responsible for holding the wedge-shaped fragment of the metacarpal in its normal relation with the articular surface of the trapezium. The essential deformity of this injury is one of angulation with the concave aspect on the volar side ; the intact soft tissues which are to act as the ' hinge ' for the reduction are thus to be found on the volar aspect of the base of the metacarpal.

Mechanics of Reduction and Fixation

It is sometimes stated that unless traction is used the reduction of this fracture cannot be held with any degree of certainty ; according to this teaching, traction is usually applied with skin adhesive attached to an outrigger built into the plaster. But as pointed out on page 50, traction is indicated only in those fractures with no inherent stability against shortening ; the Bennett's fracture, on the contrary, is one which possesses considerable potential stability and, provided that it is treated with the carpo-metacarpal joint in full extension, the reduction can always be rendered stable.

If after the reduction of a Bennett's fracture the metacarpal of the thumb is fully extended so as to tighten the volar ligaments, it becomes impossible for dorsal displacement to recur. If, now, the thumb in the reduced and extended position is slowly flexed, a critical point is reached beyond which further flexion will lever the base of the bone in a dorsal direction and so out of the joint.

Mechanical Analogy

The action of muscular tone on this reduction can be likened to the action of a crank and connecting-rod. There is a point in the motion of a crank known

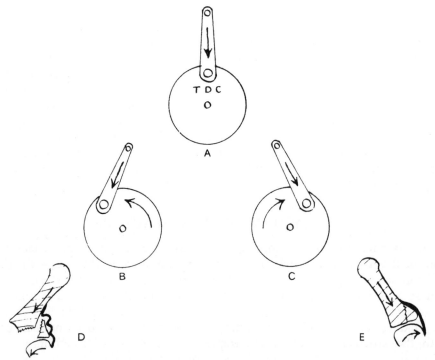

Fig. 115

Mechanical analogy in the reduction and fixation of a Bennett's fracture. The crank at 'top dead centre' A represents the position when the injury is treated by traction—the bone is in a state of uncertain equilibrium and floats without positive control. Without traction, the tone of the muscles can induce complete dislocation if the thumb is allowed to flex, B, D. Without traction, muscular tone will enhance the security of reduction if the thumb metacarpal is placed in full extension, C, E. In full extension muscular tone generates positive pressure against the undisplaced fragment.

as 'top dead centre'; on one side of this centre, pressure from the connecting-rod initiates movement in one direction of rotation (*e.g.*, towards stable reduction), while on the other side of this centre, motion will be initiated in the opposite direction (*e.g.*, towards unstable reduction) (Fig. 115). In the extended position of the metacarpal the tone of the muscles acting on the thumb will increase the stability of the reduction by thrusting the base of the bone deeper into the carpo-metacarpal socket.

144

The same mechanical analogy also explains why the use of traction is not an ideal arrangement for holding the reduction of a Bennett's fracture. Traction will merely ' float ' the base of the metacarpal in the neutral position of instability (top dead centre), whereas what is desired is the forceful impaction of the metacarpal into its socket in the absence of traction by allowing rotation to occur towards the direction of stability (Fig. 115).

TECHNIQUE

This fracture-dislocation is particularly suited to reduction under local anæsthesia, which also allows the surgeon a second attempt under the same anæsthetic if he is not satisfied with his first.

The reduction of a Bennett's fracture tests the fineness of the surgeon's sense of touch ; if approached with a heavy hand expecting a sharp click to indicate a successful reduction, it is probable that failure will result. It is no uncommon sight to see the beginner using violence on the reduction yet being uncertain that he has moved the fracture ; this is for the simple reason that a complete reduction was probably produced by the first touch of his hand but, not understanding this, the fracture is enclosed in a defective plaster and when X-rayed is then found to be unreduced.

The sensation of reduction in a Bennett's fracture is sometimes so difficult to detect that **the reduction often demands assistance from the eye to confirm the fact that the base of the thumb is in fact slipping in and out of the metacarpo-carpal joint as the reduction forces are applied and removed.** Quite often the reduction can be done without anæsthesia once the surgeon has acquired the feel of it.

To reduce the injury the metacarpal must be extended by applying pressure to the volar aspect of the *head* of the metacarpal and at the same time pressing on the dorsal surface of the base of the metacarpal. It will be noticed that traction is not an essential part of this reduction though it assists in starting the movement. If the two forces are released and the metacarpal allowed to flex, the base of the thumb will be *seen* to ride up and out of joint. It is important to repeat this movement several times till this delicate sensation is clearly recognised by *touch*, for it is by this sensation alone that reduction can be detected when the plaster has been applied. Extension of the thumb should not be too extreme, because then another mechanism seems to force the dislocation out. The best position is just short of full, forced extension.

A pad of adhesive felt is now stuck over the base of the metacarpal and the sensation of reduction by touch is again rehearsed ; the sensation will now be muffled and will need even more concentration to recognise than it did before.

A very wet plaster is now rapidly applied to hand and thumb, without any attempt to hold the reduced position. It is essential that the whole plaster should be completed while still quite soft ; if this cannot be done with proprietary quick-setting plasters it is important to use an ordinary slow-setting bandage.

With the plaster soft, wet, and complete, the surgeon now feels again for the sensation of reduction previously rehearsed; having again recognised it through wet plaster, he holds on to the position of full extension of the thumb with

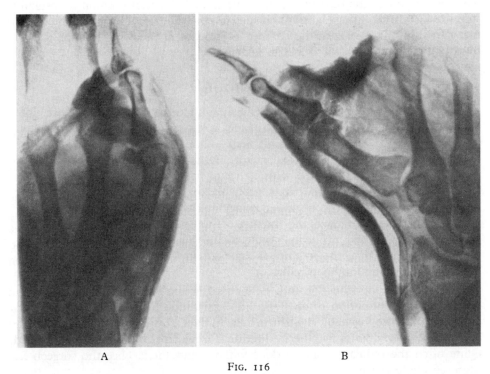

A   B

FIG. 116

A, Typical failure to reduce a Bennett's fracture because the thumb metacarpal is not fully extended.
B, Complete reduction secured when the metacarpal is fully extended at the carpo-metacarpal joint.

local pressure over the dorsum of the base of the metacarpal until the plaster is firmly set (Fig. 116).

A Common Error

A common error in performing the reduction as described above is to apply force to the volar aspect of the proximal *phalanx* instead of to the volar aspect of the *head* of the metacarpal (Fig. 117, A). **This mistake results in the metacarpophalangeal joint being extended without of necessity extending the thumb metacarpal.** In other words, the distal joints of the thumb need not be extended provided that the metacarpal is fully extended; in some people with 'double joints' extension of the distal part of the thumb is no indication of the position of the metacarpal (Fig. 118).

For this simple manipulative method to be successful it is essential that the injury should be recent. A delay of four or five days seriously prejudices the ability to hold the reduction and late slipping is very likely, and this is particularly the case if others have failed on previous attempts to reduce it.

146

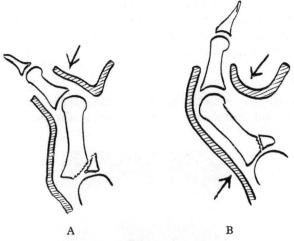

FIG. 117

Diagram illustrating a common error in the treatment of a
Bennett's fracture. A, Extension of the metacarpal is not to
be mistaken for extension at the metacarpo-phalangeal joint
in persons with undue mobility at this site. B, The plaster
must be modelled against the palmar aspect of the head of
the metacarpal as well as over the dorsal aspect of the base
of the metacarpal.

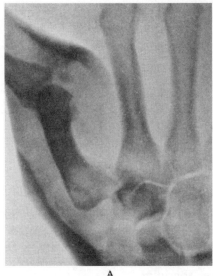
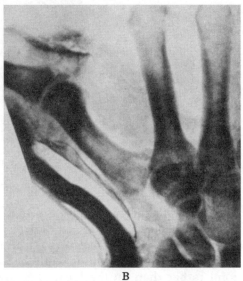

A   B

FIG. 118

A, Faulty reduction of Bennett's fracture because metacarpal is not abducted though the
metacarpo-phalangeal joint is extended.

B, Reduction secured by abducting the thumb metacarpal (the original films show complete
reduction though superficial inspection of this reproduction suggests that it is incomplete).

147

Though I have emphasised the importance of full extension of the metacarpo-carpal joint, there are some cases where extreme extension has the reverse effect. Extreme extension can force the base of the metacarpal into redislocation and a stable position of reduction may be felt just short of full extension.

Post-reduction

It is unnecessary to retain the plaster for more than four weeks. During the post-reduction period complaints of severe pain at the site of pressure over the

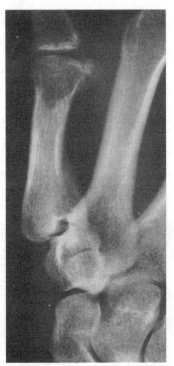

Fig. 119
Old unreduced Bennett's fracture
in labouring man which caused
no symptoms.

base of the thumb may indicate pressure necrosis of the underlying skin ; this symptom should be taken seriously lest the extensor tendon become exposed. It is never necessary to use very great pressure over the base of the thumb ; the **emphasis in the reduction should be in the extension of the carpo-metacarpal joint rather than on the local pressure over the joint.**

Unreduced Bennett's Fracture

If a Bennett's fracture is received late, or if it slips under treatment, there is no need to alarm the patient by a too pessimistic prognosis. All fixation should be abolished and active movements and gripping exercises started. A function of 75 to 90 per cent. of normal is to be expected after one or two years. The development of crippling arthritis, though theoretically possible, is not, I believe, common even with gross displacement. Fig. 119 illustrates a case in a manual worker where there was no incapacity.

In patients with osteo-arthritis at the carpo-metacarpal joint of the thumb it is the exception rather than the rule to see a mal-reduced Bennett's fracture as the cause of the arthritis. Most cases of osteo-arthritis of this joint, which is a not uncommon condition, are either cases of primary osteo-arthritis or are of osteo-arthritis superimposed on rheumatoid arthritis, and are most commonly seen in women where the traumatic origin is not likely to be present.

CHAPTER ELEVEN

FINGER FRACTURES

THE finger fracture which of all others demands most expert mechanical treatment is that of the proximal phalanx. The reputation of a surgeon may stand as much in jeopardy from this injury as from any fracture of the femur.

In the subsequent paragraphs a method is described which I believe to be of value, though it involves a rather heretical doctrine. It is important, therefore, that the spirit of this method should be fully understood because it contains a potential danger if the doctrine is misapplied.

ANATOMY OF THE FRACTURE

Fractures of the proximal phalanx are often compound, because they are so commonly the result of industrial injuries. The characteristic deformity is an angulation concave to the dorsum, and for the purpose of reduction the soft-tissue ' hinge ' is to be regarded as being on the dorsal aspect of the fracture.

Mechanics of Treatment

The reduction of these fractures as a rule offers no great difficulty; the real difficulty lies in the application of a retentive apparatus which will hold securely the reduction so easily obtained by the surgeon's fingers.

Manipulative reduction is obtained by first applying traction and hyperextension; then, with the thumb applied as a fulcrum to the volar aspect of the fracture, the traction is followed by a movement of flexion, following which the traction is released (Fig. 120). After release of the traction the reduction can be held by a simple three-point arrangement of forces designed to maintain the finger flexed over a fulcrum.

Sometimes difficulty in reduction may be experienced when the distal fragment is rotated through 90 degrees (Fig. 121, A); in these cases the method of increasing the dorsal concavity before straightening the finger will usually succeed. This procedure is so important, as a general principle, that the description is worthy of repetition, though I have described it in detail for fractures of the distal third of the femoral shaft (p. 185). With the proximal fragment held in a horizontal position the distal fragment is drawn vertically upwards to lie at right angles to it (Fig. 121, B); in this position the distal fragment is drawn powerfully upwards and the proximal fragment is pushed powerfully downwards, in the hope of getting the distal fragment to lie above the dorsal surface of the proximal; from this position the fracture is gently straightened and the fragments should then be in alignment. This step is of great value in attempting that very difficult reduction

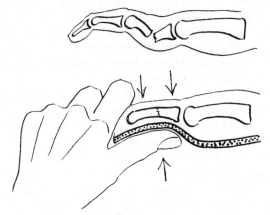

FIG. 120

Reduction of a fracture of the proximal phalanx with a three-point system of forces. Note the hold when the wet plaster slab is interposed between the surgeon's thumb and the fracture and pressure maintained until it is set.

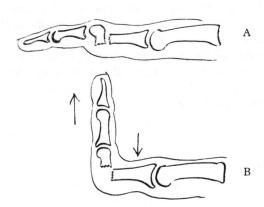

FIG. 121

Reduction of a phalangeal fracture by increasing the initial angulation and then flexing.

of the supracondylar phalangeal fracture in which there is 90 degrees of rotation of the distal fragment.

Splintage

The natural difficulty of splinting finger fractures is made even more difficult by the popular desire to leave adjacent digits free and so capable of independent movement. The use of traction is convenient because it enables a three-point system to be applied without bulky encircling dressings to impede the movement of adjacent fingers. Traction used in this way is not needed to maintain length but merely to hold the finger in contact with the curved surface of the volar splint which moulds the fracture into its correct alignment. This method can give excellent results *provided that the traction is not applied by the abominable method of transfixing the pulp of the finger with wire.* In order to prevent rotational deformity in this method it is often advised that in all fingers the traction should be directed towards the tubercle of the scaphoid.

The method to be advocated here does not employ traction. In this method **the adjacent uninjured finger is used as a splint and mould for the injured digit.** By splinting the injured finger to the adjacent normal finger the correct alignment of the fracture is automatically obtained. The fixation enforced on the adjacent normal finger enhances the immobilisation of the injured finger which is important in compound injuries.

Alignment

If an attempt be made to splint an isolated finger by a circular padded cast it is likely that two deformities will ensue, namely, angulation and rotation. In the case of the index finger radial displacement of the distal fragment may be produced because *the attempt to pass turns of bandage within the cleft between the index and the adjacent finger makes parallel alignment impossible* (Fig. 122). The other deformity likely to follow from isolated splintage of one digit is rotation. It is often said that rotational deformity can be prevented by aligning the fingers towards the tubercle of the scaphoid; but with so many other things to think about at the moment of reduction this advice is often overlooked. *If the injured finger lies side-by-side with the next normal digit, using a plaster cast which encircles both, rotary alignment cannot be lost.*

Rest

The time during which a fractured finger must be absolutely fixed need never be longer than three weeks. After this time intermittent splintage can be allowed for a further two or three weeks and then all splintage can be abandoned.

Fixation of the normal finger for three weeks can cause no permanent disability; indeed a normal finger is better capable of tolerating a period of fixation without permanent harm than is any abnormal digit.

In finger injuries the commonest cause of permanent and crippling joint stiffness can be traced to the effects of sepsis or nerve injury. In a simple finger fracture stiffness from fixation alone, in the absence of sepsis, may need weeks or months to rehabilitate, but *the ultimate prognosis is good.* By contrast, the stiffness resulting from sepsis or complicating nerve injury is permanent and irreparable. If the injured digit becomes septic its ultimate fate is largely out of the surgeon's control. The ultimate function of a septic finger will depend on how swiftly the sepsis is resolved by rest and chemotherapy.

Even more serious than sepsis localised to the injured digit is the effect of sepsis on the tendons of adjacent fingers threatening stiffness of the whole hand. It should be obvious that attempts to move a septic finger will in no way prevent stiffness of that digit. When sepsis is established in the injured digit

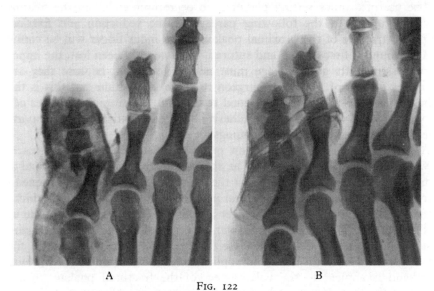

A   B

FIG. 122

A, Showing the deformity which results when a digit is splinted separately, due to the bulk of dressings interposed in the cleft between the adjacent normal digit.

B, Showing improvement in the alignment when the fractured digit and the normal adjacent digit are splinted together without bulky dressings interposed in the cleft between them. This same procedure also eliminates the danger of a rotary deformity.

attempts to keep the *normal fingers mobile* are highly to be commended. The splintage of normal and injured fingers alike is therefore only to be entertained while an open fracture is still fresh and free from sepsis ; **during the first three weeks after a compound fracture the enhanced rest enforced on the whole hand by this method may be the determining factor in preventing sepsis.** Late movement, by avoiding aggravation of sepsis, may thus result in better ultimate function than early movement. It is a grievous mistake to believe that the use of antibiotics will allow fundamental principles of surgery to be transgressed ; rest of an open wound must always be the first surgical principle and chemotherapy the second.

It will be seen from the above reasoning (1) that the complete fixation of normal fingers can do no harm *in the absence of sepsis* ; (2) that if the fracture is freshly compound the fixation of adjacent normal fingers may be the deciding factor in preventing infection.

If infection should ensue in the injured finger, encouragement of movement of adjacent fingers becomes of paramount importance. The possibility that amputation of the septic finger may eventually have to be undertaken must not be too long ignored if there is any risk of the infection impairing the mobility of adjacent normal digits.

TECHNIQUE

The use of a quick-setting plaster is to be recommended in the treatment of finger fractures. In the following paragraphs the reduction and fixation of a compound fracture of the proximal phalanx of an index finger will be considered.

The wound is first excised and sutured. If tissue has been lost, the importance of small skin grafts at this stage must not be forgotten, because they are well within the powers of a casualty surgeon to stitch in position and this is the time when they are most likely to give good results. A dressing of one layer of gauze is applied to the wound with an adhesive such as Mastisol; it is important to leave the finger free from bulky dressings.

A quick-setting plaster slab is now prepared of sufficient length to reach from the wrist to the end of the finger. The slab is folded so as to be thick and narrow in the distal part and wide and flat at the proximal part where it is fastened to the volar aspect of the wrist. In the distal part the slab should be $\frac{1}{2}$ inch thick, so as to offer a solid foundation for the finger; thin and flexible slabs are quite useless.

The wet slab is laid under the volar aspect of the digit and held against the wrist by an assistant. The surgeon seizes the distal part of the finger, together with the slab, in his right hand and applies traction. The thumb of the surgeon's right hand is applied to the volar aspect of the fractured phalanx to act as a fulcrum; the wet plaster slab thus lies between the thumb and the fracture (Fig. 120). In securing this grip it will be found that the end of the injured finger is gripped in the crook of the surgeon's index and ring fingers. The final movement of reduction is now carried out as previously described, and as though no plaster were intervening. From the position of traction and slight hyperextension the finger is flexed over the fulcrum provided by the surgeon's thumb and the traction force is then relaxed. While waiting for the plaster to set, with the surgeon's fingers still in the above position, the assistant bandages the proximal part of the slab to the wrist with circular turns of wet cotton bandage.

When the plaster has set, the surgeon releases his grip and lays the adjacent uninjured ring finger at the side of the injured digit. The dorsal aspect of both digits is now covered with wool and a gauze bandage applied *to encircle both fingers and the slab* (Fig. 123, A, B, C,). It will be seen that the injured finger is lying directly on the plaster slab without bulky dressings to interfere with the positive action of the splint as a fulcrum or mould. The plaster slab controls angulation in the sagittal plane, the adjacent finger controls lateral angulation and rotary deformity. The dorsal pad of wool keeps the finger pressed against the curved splint and permits swelling without constriction. If the wound is

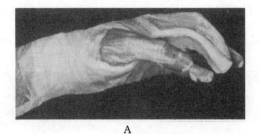

A

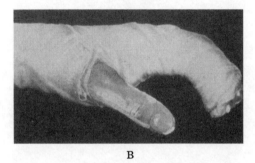

B

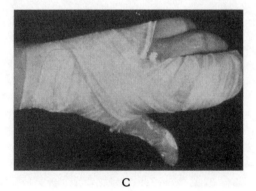

C

FIG. 123

A, Showing the palmar plaster slab used for a fracture of the proximal phalanx of the index finger. The slab is thick under the finger and has set in the position imposed on it by pressure of the surgeon's fingers.

B and C, Showing the final appearances when the adjacent normal middle finger is bandaged against the fractured digit to ensure correct alignment and to enhance the fixation.

155

sealed with a suitable adhesive dressing there should be no fear of soiling the wound with wet plaster over gauze; quick-setting proprietary plasters are practically sterile.

The radiological appearance of a fractured index finger lying side-by-side in

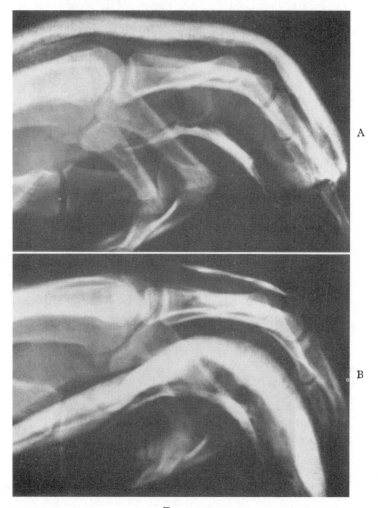

FIG. 124

Dorsal plaster slab, A, does not offer fulcrum to correct concave dorsal angulation as does palmar slab, B.

parallel alignment with the normal ring finger, and bandaged to the same volar plaster slab, is illustrated in Fig. 124, C.

The importance of using a plaster slab on the palmar aspect of the digit is illustrated in Fig. 124, A and B. In the upper figure there is slight residual angulation in the proximal fragment, concave on the dorsal aspect; the finger had been splinted with a plaster slab on the dorsal surface of the digit. Because a dorsal slab does not exert a three-point system of forces I was unhappy about this slight angulation and, though this amount of angulation in itself would be acceptable, the dorsal slab might permit this angulation to increase. I therefore changed the dorsal plaster slab to a thick *palmar* slab strong enough to act as a fulcrum under the site of angulation ; an appreciable improvement in the alignment of the fracture

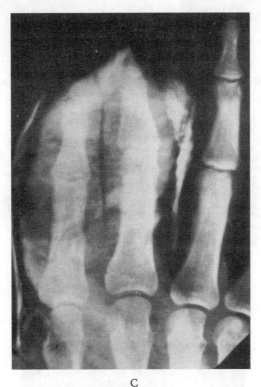

C

FIG. 124

Fractured digit plastered side-by-side with intact
digit to control later angulation.

was obtained as well as much greater certainty of maintaining this alignment (Fig. 124, B). The *thickness* of the palmar slab should be noted.

A Warning on Radiographic Control

In the treatment of finger fractures I have noticed a common error in the acceptance of post-reduction radiographs which are not true lateral views of the digit. It is often difficult to get a perfect lateral radiograph of a finger without the shadow of the adjacent finger being superimposed. For this reason, radiographers have a tendency to take oblique views so as to project the shadow of each digit separately on the film. These oblique views can be misleading and it is preferable

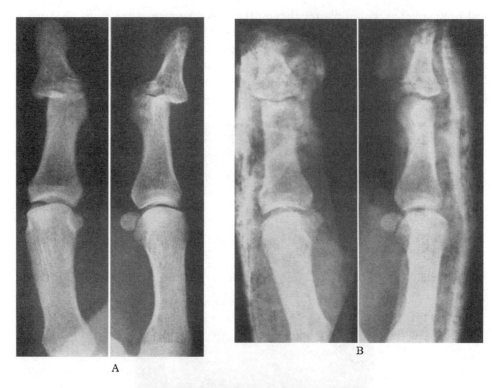

A

B

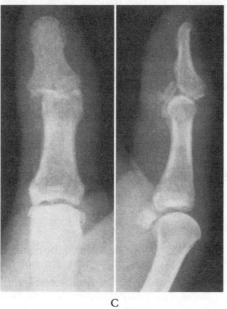

C

FIG. 125

See text for the series of technical errors leading to this bad result.

to have the shadows of two digits superimposed and attempt, even with difficulty, to trace out the appropriate shadows.

The fracture-dislocation of the terminal interphalangeal joint of a thumb shown in Fig. 125 is interesting because the errors committed illustrate some fundamental features of fracture treatment :

1. The direction of the force needed to secure any reduction is always the opposite of that causing the injury. If extension caused the injury, then flexion is needed to reduce and to hold it and vice versa.

2. The violence which caused this injury was easily elicited : during a game of football the ball which the player was holding in his hand was kicked by another player, forcing his thumb into hyperextension. The ruptured soft parts would therefore be on the palmar aspect of the joint and the intact structures in the dorsal aspect. Thus the *distal joint ought to have been splinted in flexion to tighten the dorsal structures*.

3. The final mistake was to accept a post-operative X-ray which was not perfectly centred. This is a common mistake in the handling of finger fractures because of the difficulty of getting true lateral views if other digits are superimposed. If necessary a dental film placed between the fingers should be used to settle the matter if any doubt exists.

Rehabilitation

After three weeks of fixation the finger can be started on intermittent exercise substituting the plaster with a detachable slab. The detachable plaster is discarded when test indicates that union is sound, which may take a further two to three weeks. A useful method of guarding a finger, at the same time as permitting function, is to strap it to the adjacent finger so as to leave the joints free. In gaining confidence for the early removal of splintage in finger fractures the small mechanical strains on the callus should be appreciated (p. 58). The late deformity of soft callus is related, among other factors, to the weight of the distal limb and the length of the distal fragment ; it will be readily appreciated that a finger will expose its callus to infinitely less strain than will a fracture of a femur, and therefore movement can be countenanced at a much earlier stage without the danger of spontaneous deformity.

CHAPTER TWELVE

PERTROCHANTERIC FRACTURES OF THE NECK OF THE FEMUR

IT is now universally agreed that pertrochanteric fractures of the femur are best treated by internal fixation whenever this is feasible. Because many of the patients with pertrochanteric fractures are in an advanced state of senility, sometimes complicated by mild dementia and incontinence, the non-operative treatment of these fractures presents formidable nursing difficulties.

Not all pertrochanteric fractures of the femur are suitable for internal fixation by the blade plate, and attempted operation may cause such comminution in some cases that to persist with difficult surgery is not to be advised and the case is better returned to the ward for treatment on traction. There will always be a place for the non-operative treatment of the pertrochanteric fracture, and it is necessary therefore to decide what technical matters are of importance with regard to the comfort of the patient and the convenience of the nursing staff.

RUSSELL TRACTION

It is obvious that some form of balanced traction is the only rational method of non-operative treatment, because a plaster hip-spica is quite out of the question in patients of this degree of senility. The most generally used type of traction is that popularly known as Russell traction. In its original form Russell devised this system for the treatment of fractures of the *shaft* of the femur and he evolved the rather complicated system of pulleys in order to correlate the traction force necessary to maintain length with the *upward lifting force necessary to correct backward angulation at the fracture*. To do this the fracture was supported in a sling under the distal third of the thigh, and the traction force was attached to the sling to give an upward lift by an arrangement of pulleys (Fig. 132, c). The same cord dispensing the traction force passed, in its course to the weight, through pulleys which doubled its effective pull and exerted this product in the length of the tibia below the knee. By estimating the direction of the traction force acting on the sling a parallelogram of force could be worked out and the resultant force acting in the axis of the femur could be calculated.

In the treatment of pertrochanteric fractures by Russell traction the original complicated system of pulleys is really quite unnecessary. Reduced to its mechanical elements all that is required is a means of suspending the lower extremity and a means of applying traction in the axis of the femur. For pertrochanteric fractures there is no need for the two forces to be correlated in any subtle fashion because there is no need for an upward lift to correct the backward angulation present in a shaft fracture.

The Importance of Skeletal Traction

To secure good results in the way most comfortable for the patient and most convenient for the nursing staff, skeletal traction applied to the tibial tubercle is incomparably better than adhesive traction. **Adhesive traction should always be avoided in combination with weight traction.** Weight traction on skin adhesive almost inevitably results in a 'creeping' of the adhesive strapping, pressure sores are produced, excoriation of the skin is frequent, and pain is invariable. External popliteal paralysis is a frequent result of adhesive traction, because, as it slides down the leg week by week, it carries the circular turns of cotton bandage which surround it and these constrict the limb as they pass from the small circumference at the level of the knee to the larger circumference near the head of the fibula. **Adhesive skin traction is to be recommended only in conjunction with fixed traction.** Fixed traction force on skin adhesive can only be temporarily excessive, because the adhesive slips or stretches until the tension falls again to a tolerable level and thereafter, unlike weight traction, no further slipping will take place. The misery which can result from weight traction applied to adhesive strapping is great enough in the young adult, but when applied to the senile case with its papery, inelastic skin and general low vitality, the result is often most distressing. The failure to use skeletal traction in these old people, and the choice of skin adhesive, arises from a misplaced feeling that skeletal traction is a drastic measure which they might be unable to stand. But a Steinmann nail can be inserted under local anæsthetic in the ward and at the bedside with the greatest ease, and all the patient's discomfort is thereafter at an end.

TECHNIQUE

Having inserted a Steinmann nail into the tibial tubercle, it is strongly to be recommended that the surgeon should apply a below-knee plaster cast, *over adequate padding*, and **incorporating the Steinmann nail in the upper end of the plaster.** In this way *a traction unit* is constructed as described on page 180. Having completed the traction unit, it can be suspended from a Balkan beam and a 10 lb. traction weight, arranged to give a horizontal pull by means of cords and pulleys (Fig. 126). *The incorporation of the Steinmann nail in the upper end of the plaster is specially stressed because of the danger of external popliteal paralysis if the upper end of the plaster is left loose and capable of cutting into the limb.*

The Denham nail is a great improvement over the original Steinmann nail in the treatment of old people in whom the bone of the tibial tubercle is osteoporotic. In this type of bone the Steinmann nail rapidly becomes loose and then starts to slide sideways and ulceration of the skin is brought about. The Denham nail (Fig. 127) is provided with a short length of screw thread positioned slightly to the side of the middle which is nearest the end gripped by the introducer. This short length of thread engages with the lateral cortex of the tibia and holds the nail securely against medial and lateral slipping.[1]

[1] I do not recommend this nail for use in compression arthrodesis. In order to manufacture this nail it has to be of much softer metal than that of the ordinary 4 mm. Steinmann nail which is work-hardened in the wire-drawing process. Under high pressures the Denham nail will pass the elastic limit and fail to operate as a spring and the screw thread, acting as a ' stress raiser,' may induce fatigue fracture under the conditions of compression arthrodesis.

A satisfactory method of suspending the traction unit is illustrated in Fig. 126. A plaster loop is incorporated in the plaster to facilitate attachment of a cord to the foot of the cast. Two pulleys are arranged on the Balkan beam

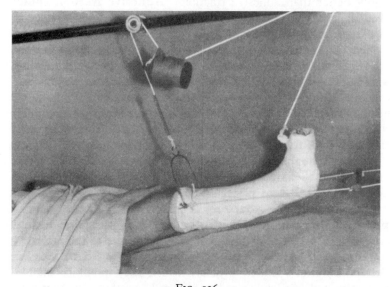

FIG. 126

Modified Russell traction for pertrochanteric fractures—using the pin-and-plaster traction unit. The whole limb should be strongly abducted.

2 feet apart and a cord is passed over them to suspend the cast. The length of this cord should be such that there is no slack when the leg is held out with the knee straight and almost touching the surface of the bed (Fig. 128, A). A weight of about 7 lb. is now attached to the horizontal part of the cord *close to the pulley*

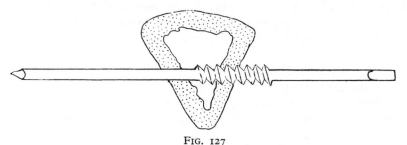

FIG. 127

Denham nail. Particularly suitable for holding skeletal traction in the porous bones of elderly patients for two or three months without loosening.

which is nearest the head of the patient. *This weight must not be loose on the cord but must be rigidly tied into the cord.* This detail ensures that there is more upward lift on the knee than there is on the foot, so that the leg does not always lie with the knee fully extended. The patient can raise the leg with the knee straight (Fig. 128, B) and then flex the knee (Fig. 128, C). To permit knee movements the

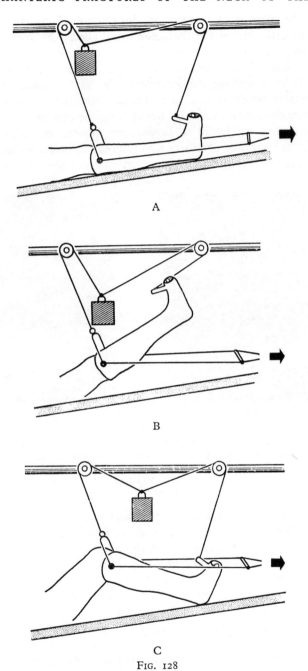

A

B

C

FIG. 128

Mechanical arrangement of Russell traction. Overhead
weight is fixed to the cord (not sliding on the cord) and
attached nearer to knee than foot, A, in order to elevate
knee more than foot.

cords carrying the main traction force in the horizontal direction to their point of attachment to each end of the Steinmann nail should be kept wide apart with a wooden spreader.

Padding the Heel.—It is important to take the greatest care with the padding of the heel. Felt or sponge rubber should be placed under the heel before applying the plaster which is needed to prevent equinus. If wool alone is used there is still some danger of pressure sores despite the plaster.

In no circumstances should a below-knee plaster be used over adhesive traction; the danger of pressure sores is very great and the combination of plaster of Paris and adhesive traction should be regarded as an abomination.

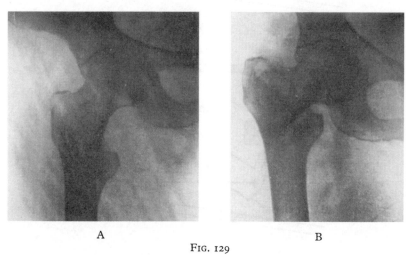

A   B

FIG. 129

A, Pertrochanteric fracture while on traction and over-distracted as shown by slight valgus position. This delays consolidation and encourages, B, collapse into coxa vara even as late as three months after the injury.

Post-operative

Having established this traction system and having placed the limb in some degree of abduction, the further conduct of the case is quite straightforward, and there is little else which is not obvious on common-sense grounds. One fact only needs mentioning, and that is a warning that these fractures are very prone to the late development of coxa vara unless the traction is maintained for a minimum of twelve weeks. Even after this time some recurrence of this deformity is possible, due undoubtedly to the collapse of the fracture into the cavity in the cancellous bone left when the fracture has been disimpacted under the traction force (Fig. 129 and Figs. 10 and 11, pp. 10 and 11). Too much correction of the deformity in the direction of coxa valga is therefore not to be recommended, and the acceptance of a slight degree of coxa vara from the outset is advisable in the interests of rapid consolidation. Even after three months the collapse of the fracture under partial weight-bearing is very likely, and therefore weight-bearing should be postponed for at least six months. The tendency to late deformity in this fracture is another reason why the internal fixation of this fracture by the blade plate is steadily gaining general favour. Some idea of the enormous forces available to produce coxa vara, even in the later stages of treatment, can be drawn from the fact that blade plates can fracture during the period of early rehabilitation.

Used in the manner described, the comfort of these aged patients is quite surprising, and it will be seen that the non-operative method is far from being the lethal procedure which some enthusiasts of the blade plate proclaim it to be. The high mortality which is associated with the conservative method is the result of continuous pain and discomfort which wears out these old people ; on skeletal traction these old patients become happy and their health is correspondingly improved. In institutions which cater for large numbers of these old patients, and when the home conditions render it impossible to receive them back unless fully ambulant, the non-operative method can hold its own against the operative, for there is no point in operating unless the relatives can take the patient home within a few weeks.

CHAPTER THIRTEEN

FRACTURES OF THE SHAFT OF THE FEMUR

THE treatment of fractures of the shaft of the femur is of particular interest, demonstrating as it does certain fundamental fracture mechanics previously described in more general terms. It seems probable that new operative methods of treating the fractured femur—such as the medullary nail of Kuntscher—will in the future take precedence over closed methods for transverse fractures of the shaft (which are always difficult to handle by conservative means) and for most other fractures in the middle and upper thirds. For fractures of the femur **in the distal third** which have been successfully reduced I believe that Thomas' method is unrivalled.

One of the many lessons we can learn from this fracture is the danger of becoming too much engrossed in minutiæ, if by so doing we lose the broad view of a problem. This is an error into which the tempo of modern life makes it easy to fall. We must never lose sight of two facts : firstly, that a fracture of the shaft of a femur can often be the easiest of fractures to treat conservatively ; and secondly, that *full recovery* after a fracture of the femur takes about one year (which is the time necessary for full reconstruction of the ivory shaft of this bone). These are facts which we tend to forget when assessing new methods which apparently offer quick dividends and short hospitalisation. *Procedures adopted in the early phases of treatment can sometimes have disappointing and unexpected repercussions at a later date.* Thus in the case of early knee movement during the treatment of a fracture of the femur a considerable range of knee movement at three months is easily obtained in many traction-suspension methods, but if bony union is present only as a precarious bridge, or if fibrous union results, the need for a plaster hip-spica or a caliper splint may completely negate the early prospects of full knee range. **In some cases early knee movement may be responsible for fibrous union of the fracture, and hence a stiffer knee may result than if no joint exercise had been permitted in the early phases.** In the same way concentration on early knee movement may invite the appearance of a late varus deformity because this is difficult to prevent in any apparatus allowing knee movement. To end with the visible deformity of bow leg is but poor compensation for a good range of knee movement ; this is all the more unfortunate when it is realised that a straight leg could in all probability have been secured by a slower method and still with a serviceable range of knee movement.

It is not out of place here to comment on a strange fact ; while a patient will blame his surgeon for late deformity, he will usually tend to blame himself for knee stiffness. A patient regards deformity as something completely within the surgeon's scope, but often thinks that knee stiffness arises from defective material with which the surgeon has had to contend. If there exists deformity as well as knee stiffness, the patient invariably connects the two and explains the knee stiffness quite simply—' because the surgeon never " set " the leg properly ! '

Remote repercussions of early treatment on late results must also be considered in the operative treatment of fractures of the femur just as much as in the non-operative methods. If we see a case demonstrating the merits of internal fixation, we must first ascertain whether this result could also have followed the simplest form of conservative treatment (as is often the case in oblique or spiral fractures). If the operation of plating is favoured on the theory that it will facilitate early knee movement, it must not be forgotten that callus production is thereby commonly inhibited ; and if callus is tardy in its appearance the plate may angulate and the slow consolidation may result in a permanent restriction of knee movement through the need for late fixation in hip-spica or bone grafting ; thus the end result is the very opposite of what was intended.

Nor must the dangers of sepsis be lightly dismissed in the internal fixation of fractures of the shaft of the femur. *A solitary instance of sepsis in any series should be regarded as considerably reducing the merit of the series as a whole.* Sepsis after the plating of a femur is possible, because the operation often demands considerable muscular exertion from the surgeon, may consume much time, and may necessitate a very extensive exposure of the shaft. The operation is usually required in athletic young adults where the retraction of bulky investing muscles offers considerable difficulty. **Sepsis is the commonest single cause of permanent joint stiffness, and it must not be forgotten that an infection which resolves on chemotherapy may still scar the muscle of the quadriceps with serious consequences for knee movement.** One cannot help suspecting that some cases which run temperatures after operation, but which never discharge pus, may fall into this category.

Viewed in its broadest aspects, the problem of the fractured femur has no simple solution by conservative means, nor can any simple dictum be enunciated to guide the inexperienced. It is an over-simplification to say that the problem of the fractured femur is the problem of the stiff knee ; quite as great a problem is the late deformity (varus bowing), which is the ugly penalty of concentrating too much on early knee movement. **A good conservative result is a successful compromise between minimum deformity and minimum restriction of joint movement.** A good conservative method is one which yields a constant satisfactory result rather than a series of perfect cases interspersed with an odd catastrophe.

The healing of the fractured femur must be regarded as a process extending over a twelve-month period ; this is the time taken for the complete reconstruction of the cortex of the femoral shaft. First and foremost this fracture is a fracture of a weight-bearing bone ; it is also a fracture of a bone which possesses long levers, thereby exposing the callus to abnormally high stresses. The soundest plan of treatment is that which is directed primarily to securing sound bony union in the shortest possible time; this can only be done by planning to eliminate all factors which are known to delay consolidation. My own experience leads me to believe that **if sound bony union can be secured in three months, there will be an excellent recovery of knee movement by the end of one year even if no movement of the joint is permitted in the early months of treatment.**

It is the purpose of the following pages to attempt to expound the opinion

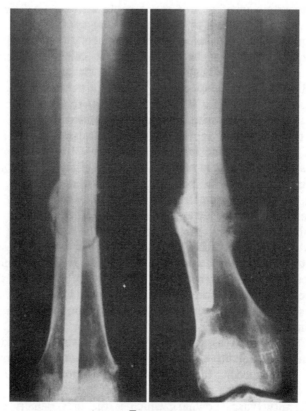

FIG. 130

Showing how intramedullary nail cannot control angulation in lower third of femoral shaft unless nail is passed so far distally as almost to penetrate knee joint.

that, *for fracture in the lower third of the shaft of the femur*, the conservative treatment using the Thomas splint is superior to all other methods, either operative or non-operative. From being, as it is in some circles, relegated to the status of a crude first-aid device, it is hoped to show that the Thomas splint possesses mechanical features which are superior to any other closed method, and that it is superior to any of the operative methods which use plates, because the latter may impede the mobility of muscles which have such a large excursion in relation to the lower third of the shaft. In the *lower third* of the femur the intramedullary nail by itself is not satisfactory because the expanding lumen of the distal fragment offers but a poor hold for the nail (Fig. 130). In fractures of the *middle third* the method of Thomas is unsuitable as a method of choice because the control of the proximal fragment is uncertain. The intramedullary nail would appear to be almost an ideal solution at the *midshaft*, as in the *upper third*.

Deformity

Classical fractures have classical deformities. Deformities are of two kinds : initial and late. Initial deformities result from the balance of muscle groups acting on the fragments ; late deformities often depend on the method used for the treatment of the fracture. Late deformities are not necessarily the same as initial deformities ; thus in the lower third of the femur the initial deformity is a backward angulation of the lower fragment, but the commonest late deformity is a varus (bow leg) angulation.

In the treatment of a fractured femur popular opinion always seems to stress the prime importance of correcting backward angulation, while the correction of varus deformity seems to be regarded as a simple matter to be dealt with *secundum artem*. In practice some residual backward angulation (though it need never occur with the Thomas method) is the least important deformity, because backward angulation can be compensated by flexion of the knee and the convex bulge of the quadriceps muscle conceals concavity in the femur. An extreme example of this is shown in the untreated femur of a native in Fig. 131, where the only disability was 2 inches of shortening and some limitation of terminal flexion (strangely enough there was no excessive hyperextension in the knee joint). By contrast a **slight varus deformity will result in an ugly bow leg if it is as much as 10 degrees, because deformity in the varus-valgus plane cannot be compensated at the knee joint and is always fully revealed when the knee is extended.** The concealment of varus deformity by the flexed position of the knee is a common reason for its presence in the end result when femurs are treated with the knee flexed to 45 degrees as they are

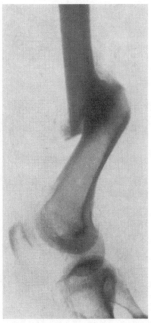

FIG. 131

Untreated femur in a native illustrating the fact that backward angulation is not a very noticeable deformity when the quadriceps fills up the anterior concavity and the knee joint compensates by flexing. Varus or valgus deformities, on the other hand, cannot be concealed, and both produce ugly appearances.

on weight-traction ; in this type of apparatus a varus bow is often noticed only on X-ray examination, whereas, had the limb been treated on the straight Thomas splint, even 5 degrees of varus bowing would have been detected at a glance.

A COMPARISON OF THE MECHANICS OF DIFFERENT
CONSERVATIVE METHODS

The method of H. O. Thomas uses fixed traction with counter-traction by the ring of the splint and stands in sharp contrast to all other conservative methods which use weight-traction with counter-traction from body weight. The methods using weight-traction, conveniently grouped under the term traction-suspension methods, are numerous but *essentially the splint takes second place to the action of*

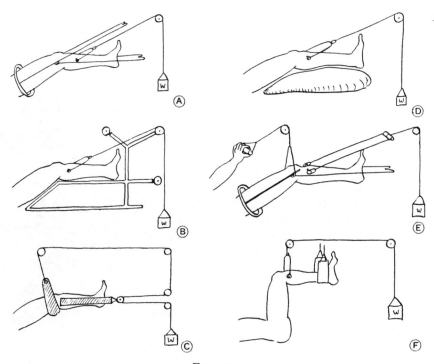

FIG. 132
Various modes of sliding traction.

the traction force, and indeed in some cases no splint is used at all. The principal modes of using weight-traction are represented by the following selection (Fig. 132) :

(A) *Thomas Splint and Pearson Knee-flexion Piece.*—Here the Thomas splint acts merely as a cradle ; it bears no fixed relation to the skeleton and can have no positive action in controlling deformity.

(B) *Braun Frame.*—This splint is again merely a cradle for the limb ; an added disadvantage is that the position of the pulleys cannot be altered and the size of the splint often does not fit the limb as exactly as might be wished. Lateral bowing is common because the splint and the distal fragment are fixed to the frame while the patient and proximal fragment can move sideways leaving the frame behind.

(C) *Russell Traction*.—Posterior angulation of the distal fragment is controlled by a sling; the lifting force of this sling is related to the main traction force through the medium of pulleys. No rigid splintage is used in this method.

(D) *Perkins*.—Here no splintage at all is used; the posterior angulation of the thigh is controlled by a pillow; alignment and fixation depend entirely on the action of continuous traction.

(E) *Fisk*.—Here an ingenious hinged version of the Thomas splint is arranged to allow 90 degrees of knee movement; it is particularly attractive in that it allows of active extension of the knee joint. Fixation and alignment depend entirely on the weight-traction and the splint merely applies the motive power for assisted knee movements.

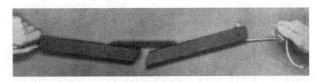

FIG. 133

Showing how traction in the axis of the femoral shaft cannot correct backward angulation but merely results in distraction with deformity persisting.

(F) ' 90—90—0.'—Here the thigh is suspended in the vertical plane by weight-traction pulling vertically upwards; the ill-effect of gravity as the cause of backward angulation of the fragments is thus eliminated.

Nearly all methods which depend on heavy traction are open to the following criticisms :

1. The action of continuous traction is frequently made to subserve a threefold function : to maintain length, preserve alignment, and fix the fragments. **It is impossible to diminish the traction force alone without jeopardising the stability of the reduction.**

2. **Gravity is not used to help in correcting the deformity of backward angulation.** The thigh, being suspended at its distal end, shows a natural tendency to sag at the fracture site under the action of gravity; this has to be combated by slings or pads which continually require adjustment.

3. There is always a tendency for the line of traction to pull into the axis of the femur. It should be an axiom that **backward angulation of the distal fragment can never be corrected by traction in the axis of the femur ;** traction in the axis merely results in elongation without correction of angulation (Fig. 133). To correct backward angulation it is necessary for the traction force to act against a rigid fulcrum placed below the distal fragment; to do this *the direction of the traction must be deflected away from the axis of the femur* so as to exert a turning movement on the lower fragment round the fulcrum (Fig. 134).

THE THOMAS METHOD

If any one maxim can ensure success by the Thomas method perhaps it is that **the fracture must always be amenable to manipulative reduction**

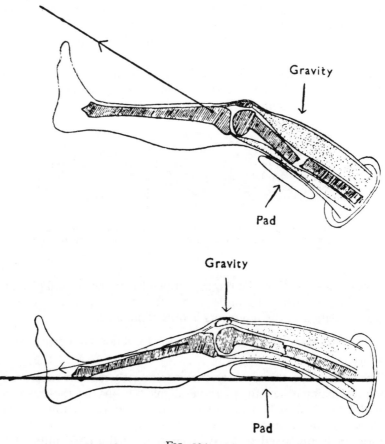

FIG. 134

Showing how gravity tends to encourage sagging at the fracture site in traction-suspension methods, but encourages anterior bowing in the Thomas method and is assisted in this by traction directed away from the axis of the femur (*i.e.*, in the axis of the tibia).

before the splint is applied. The Thomas splint with fixed traction is only capable of *maintaining* a reduction previously secured by manipulation. A common source of failure with this method arises from continuous attempts to secure additional length by repeatedly tightening the traction cords after an unsuccessful attempt at manipulative reduction.

When a fracture has been successfully reduced and has been fixed in a Thomas splint the tension in the apparatus, on recovery from the anæsthetic, should be merely that generated by the tone of the resting muscles. This method therefore differs fundamentally from traction-suspension methods where the tension in the apparatus is always that of the imposed weight and may have no relation to the physiological requirements of the muscles. Under weight-traction the ' stretch-reflex ' calls out further contraction from the muscles, and until the muscles lose their tone from fatigue or adaptation the initial weight is in excess of that demanded by the resting muscles. **With fixed traction it is the length which remains constant,** while there is a continuous diminution of traction force as the tone of the muscles diminishes, as no further stimuli are thrown in to evoke a stretch reflex. **With weight-traction it is the tension which remains constant** and the length depends on the amount of tearing of the inter-muscular septa and fibrous tissues of the thigh. *With fixed traction the fracture can be ' set ' at a predetermined length irrespective of the tone of the muscles or the laxity of soft parts.*

In the Thomas method it is undesirable to be continually re-tightening the traction cords if the length of the limb is adequate. The evidence of the tape measure is not to be despised—it is almost as helpful as the X-ray and more easily carried out.

If the fracture is oblique, adequate length can always be held with quite gentle traction. If the fracture is transverse this method possesses the desirable feature, not present in any other, that it allows the traction force to be deliberately decreased, once the bone ends have been ' hitched ' by manipulation, without invoking angulation ; because **alignment is controlled by the splint and not by the traction force.** If the fracture is transverse and manipulation has not secured a reduction, then the fracture is unsuited to this method ; in this case one may resort to open reduction.

The case illustrated in Fig. 135 is a good example of the management of a case by the Thomas method using the principle of ' controlled collapse.' *The features of special interest are :*

1. The patient was seventy-one years of age.

2. Gentle traction held the length with a predetermined amount of shortening ($\frac{1}{2}$ inch).

3. The side bars of the Thomas splint controlled the angulation in the presence of only a token traction force (not more than 2 to 3 lb.).

4. Union was facilitated by the ' controlled collapse.'

5. The first signs of clinical union were detected six weeks after the injury because fixation was incomplete ; thus active movements were possible inside the confines of the splint and the limb could easily be released to test for union.

6. Clinical union being detected, all splintage was abandoned and the limb laid over a pillow for another two weeks. If the fracture had been transverse this would not have been permissible because late angulation would be threatened, but it was safe in an oblique fracture.

7. Eight weeks after the fracture the patient had nearly 90 degrees range of movement in the knee and was permitted to take weight on the leg with assistance.

8. At four months the patient had recovered with a full range of knee movement.

Contrast this with what might easily have happened on ' balanced ' weight-traction if used by a surgeon unaware of the potential dangers of the method :

1. In order to maintain alignment, adequate tension would have to be maintained in the fascial structures of the thigh, which would necessitate 10 to 15 lb. of longitudinal traction.

2. This amount of traction would have pulled the fracture out to full length (and might even have distracted it).

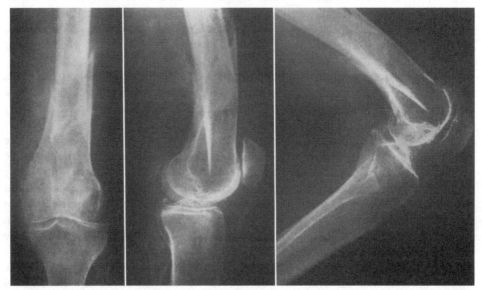

FIG. 135

Lower-third fracture of femoral shaft in patient seventy-one years of age, treated with Thomas splint, skin-extension, controlled collapse, and mobilisation as soon as clinical tests suggested union. Note flexion range (100 degrees) three months after injury. Excessive traction might have delayed consolidation.

3. Failure to promote collapse would have impaired rapid consolidation of the fracture and rendered it unsuitable for weight-bearing.

4. By using balanced traction 30 degrees of active knee movement might have been achieved at three weeks, but if consolidation had been imperfect the later progress of knee range would have been slow.

5. Attempts to diminish the amount of weight-traction would have encouraged angular deformity by allowing the fascial structures in the thigh to become slack.

If treated in a plaster cylinder or hip-spica the disadvantages would be :

1. Shortening might become excessive.

2. Fixation would be more rigid than is necessary.

3. It would be impossible to detect the first signs of the return of active movement as an indication of early union. Plaster thus would have to be retained

for an empirical period, *i.e.*, eight to twelve weeks, and thereafter rehabilitation would have to start from zero.

The Correction of Posterior Angulation

In the correction of backward angulation in fractures of the distal third of the femur the method of Thomas presents some particularly attractive features. It must be mentioned that the method to be advocated here is not exactly that described by Thomas himself; it differs from his original description in that the knee is elevated in front of the side bars of the splint by means of a large pad under the lower fragment and popliteal fossa, which causes the knee to be flexed by about 20 degrees (Fig. 136, A). In the classical description the knee was flexed by not more than 5 degrees, and it lay between the bars of the splint with two-thirds

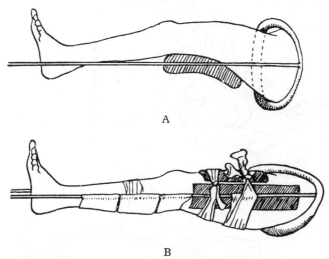

A

B

Fig. 136

A, Modified Thomas method as advocated by the writer; the whole thigh lies in front of the side bars, not two-thirds in front and one-third behind as in the original method.

B, Classical arrangement of Thomas splint as used by H. O. Thomas—reproduced from his *Contributions*.

of the knee in front and one-third behind (Fig. 136, B). With the knee straight the traction force acts only in the length of the femoral shaft and, as was posed as a maxim in a preceding paragraph, traction in the axis of the femoral shaft cannot help in the correction of backward angulation. It is probable that as used by Thomas some slight posterior angulation might often have persisted by this method, for it must be remembered that the work of Thomas preceded the X-ray. This serves to emphasise how a slight posterior angulation need cause no noticeable external deformity.

In the modified method here to be described the large pad behind the lower fragment acts as a fulcrum over which the backward angulation is corrected by the traction force. The direction of the traction force lies in the axis of the *tibia, i.e.,* 20 degrees away from the axis of the femur; the higher the pad, and therefore **the more flexed the knee, the more effective becomes the correction of backward angulation by traction in the axis of the tibia.**

It will be observed in this method how economically the force of gravity is

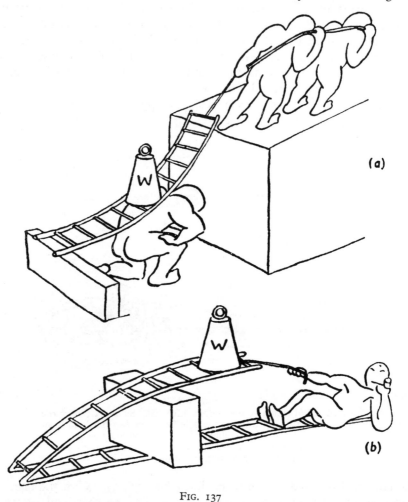

FIG. 137

Cartoon illustrating the essential difference between traction-suspension methods and the Thomas method. In the former there is a wasteful use of force to combat the ill-effects of gravity, in the latter gravity is harnessed and results in great economy of traction force and less danger of over-distraction.

coerced into restoring anterior convexity to the shaft of the femur. Instead of the fractured shaft sagging under the action of gravity by being suspended from its distal end, as it is in traction-suspension methods, the shaft is moulded over the convex surface of the pad by the weight of the thigh assisted by the pull in the length of the shaft of the tibia. This arrangement is illustrated in the cartoon in Fig. 137.

Counterpoising the Thomas Splint

The principal disadvantage in using the Thomas splint with fixed traction is that it can be very uncomfortable. The compact 'triangulated' arrangement of the forces, with the splint and pressure pad in a fixed location in regard to the limb, depends on firm contact between the padded ring of the splint and the root of the limb. If the nursing staff is not diligent in caring for the skin under the ring, this is likely to blister if fixed traction of more than a few pounds is being exerted through it. To ease the pressure of the ring against the perineum the Thomas splint, with its fixed traction *in situ*, can be counterpoised from a Balkan beam and light weight-traction can be applied to the end of the splint to keep the ring pressure comfortable (Fig. 142, p. 182). It is rarely necessary to apply a traction weight of more than 5 lb. because the fracture has already been reduced by manipulation. After the first two weeks it is often unnecessary to have any weight-traction acting in a longitudinal direction and then the fracture is merely resting on a counterpoised splint held to an adequate length by the fixed traction inside the splint.

The Thomas Splint

In its original form the ring of the splint consisted of a simple geometrical ovoid, and this is still the best shape of ring. The numerous attempts to 'improve' it, by innovations such as introducing a V-shaped dip with the idea of improving the ischial bearing, are valueless. The idea that the ring exerts its counter-extension against the tuber ischii is a fallacy which should be boldly exposed; in actual practice **the major part of the counter-extension is taken against the perineum and the fatty folds of the buttock.** To insist that the ring should exert its counter-extension only against the tuber ischii, *which it most palpably does not,* is one of the reasons why critical observers have viewed this method with distrust. H. O. Thomas in his own description of the method never uses the term tuber ischii, nor does he indicate by any other name that the ring bears against any bony point of the pelvis. Throughout his work he refers to the ring as the 'groin ring' and busies himself with the accurate fitting of the ring to the circumference of the 'root of the limb.'

Particularly objectionable are those first-aid splints which possess only a half ring, completed in front by a strap; in this type of splint the half ring is sometimes hinged to the side bars, which is a most undesirable feature except in first-aid work.

There should be a complete stock of these splints with rings varying from 11 to 26 inches in 2 inch steps. The rings should all be newly covered with soft leather and should be dressed with saddle soap. The hard, dry, cracked rings which result from previous use on other patients are not to be tolerated. An arrangement should be made with the splint shop for recovering dirty, used, rings and keeping the stock series complete. A ring should be chosen which fits the thigh as closely as possible, but it will always be found that it becomes looser as the thigh shrinks; when this occurs a pad placed between the lateral part of the ring and the great trochanter will keep the medial part of the ring from the anus and nearer to the region of the tuber ischii. *After six weeks, when the fracture is first examined for the progress of union, the splint must be changed for one with a closer fitting ring.*

The Slings

Slings should be of strong calico or flannel and should be 6 inches in width. They should be applied as illustrated in Fig. 138 so that four thicknesses are

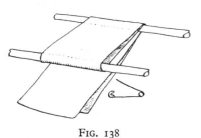

FIG. 138

Method of applying the master sling behind the lower fragment.

under the limb. The most important sling is that which supports the pad under the distal fragment—the 'master sling'; this should never be held by paper clips but **must be rigidly fixed to the side bars because it is the key to the reduction.**

A source of mechanical failure with the Thomas splint is a tendency of the master sling to slide on the side bars of the Thomas splint and so to drift away from the position initially set by the surgeon. This is easily remedied by the simple expedient of binding the side bars with adhesive strapping for a short distance before applying the master sling.

The Pad

Lying on the master sling is the pad used to support the lower fragment and popliteal fossa. The pad is made by enclosing cotton wool in a length of 6 inches diameter stockinet and turning in the ends. When compressed between the hands the pad should measure approximately 2 inches in thickness, 6 inches in width, and about 9 inches in length. It is placed transversely across the splint under the distal fragment and popliteal fossa.

Fixed Skeletal Traction

In the classical method of applying fixed traction on the Thomas splint skin traction was always used. Skin traction is uncomfortable and some patients find that itching of the skin can be greater torment than the discomfort of the fracture. Unless a nursing staff is available skilled in supervising this type of treatment, there is a great danger of pressure sores near the tendo Achillis. Paralysis of the external popliteal nerve is a not infrequent complication of skin traction on a Thomas splint, due I think to the tendency of the leg to roll into external rotation, which is difficult to check by skin traction. In the externally rotated position the external popliteal nerve moves from its normal posterolateral position in the upper part of the calf to lie directly posterior on the splint under the full weight of the leg, trapped between the slings below and the neck of the fibula above.

I do not advise the use of skin traction as primary treatment for a fresh fracture of the shaft of the femur in a strong young adult, because time may be wasted while the fracture is capable of reduction by the more positive force of skeletal traction. Experience with skin traction is of great value, however, in teaching the surgeon how easily some fractures of the femur can be kept at full length, and even distracted, by very small forces ; experience such as this fosters respect for skeletal traction.

The method of using fixed skeletal traction which I recommend combines a Steinmann nail in the tibial tuberosity with a light below-knee plaster cast. This combination of nail and plaster is what I have called a traction unit (Fig. 126, p. 162) and it offers the following features :

1. The foot is supported at right angles to the tibia.
2. The external popliteal nerve and calf muscles are protected from pressure against the slings of the splint. The tibia is suspended from the Steinmann nail inside the plaster so that an air space develops under the tibia as the calf muscles lose their bulk.
3. External rotation of the foot and distal fragment of the femur is controlled.
4. The tendo Achillis is protected from pressure sores.
5. Comfort : the patient is unaware of the traction when applied through the medium of a nail.

The traction unit is applied before starting the reduction and after threading the Thomas splint over the limb. This has to be done after the anæsthetic has been started and it takes about ten minutes to complete because the plaster must harden before it is possible to proceed with the manipulative reduction.

A Steinmann nail is passed through the tibial tuberosity and a stirrup attached. The leg is held by assistants holding the stirrup and the foot and, after applying plenty of padding around the malleoli and heel, a light below-knee plaster is applied. The plaster must incorporate the nail ; this is an important detail because unless this is done, the top edge of the plaster will cut into the calf as it lies on the Thomas splint.

A small refinement is added at this point, and though it may seem a little fussy, it will later prove of great value ; a piece of wood is applied transversely across the sole of the foot about its mid point and is incorporated in the plaster. This piece of wood should be about 6 inches in length and it rests on the side bars of the splint, so that it prevents rotation of the foot ; if desired it is possible to make the foot rest in about 10 degrees of external rotation by a suitable inclination of the cross-piece to the long axis of the foot (Fig. 139).

When the plaster of the traction unit has set, the fracture is reduced, using the Steinmann stirrup to exert powerful manual traction. During the manipulation the splint will carry only the master sling and its pressure pad to give a fulcrum for the manipulation. When the surgeon is satisfied that 'hitching' of the bone ends has been obtained, and that telescoping no longer occurs, the reduction is held by tying traction cords *to each end of the Steinmann nail* and passing them down the length of the splint, where they are tied to the end of the splint. The stirrup is not used for attaching the traction cords.

The thigh at this stage is supported by the pressure pad on the master sling, and the foot is supported by the transverse wooden bar attached to the sole of the plaster

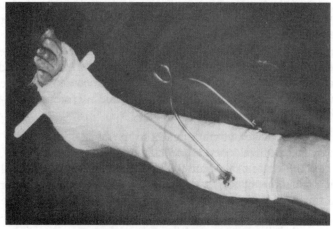

FIG. 139

Showing pin-and-plaster traction unit as an alternative to traction by adhesive plaster arranged for the treatment of a fracture of the shaft of the femur on the Thomas splint.

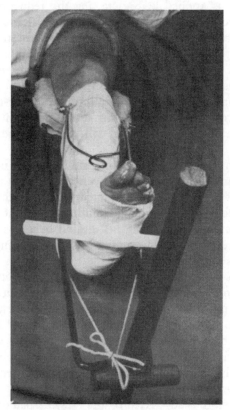

FIG. 140

Showing the function of the cross-bar fixed to the sole of the plaster traction unit. Any degree of rotation of the foot can be maintained by the position of the cross-bar.

traction unit (Fig. 140). This arrangement exposes the lower fragment to the maximum 'turning movement' to correct backward angulation, but at the same time it exposes the soft parts behind the thigh to maximum compression against the pressure pad. This compression is the sum of the weight of the limb, plus the weight of the plaster, plus a downward component of the fixed traction force. This compression can be controlled by passing a sling under the upper end of the plaster of the traction unit and tightening it until it is judged that excessive pressure has been relieved from the back of the thigh. The importance of this detail is often overlooked and in order to emphasise it this sling might be called the 'moderator sling' because it moderates the pressure of the master sling. It will be realised

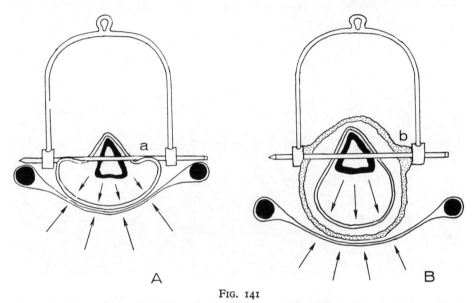

FIG. 141

Illustrating the danger of resting the leg on the slings of a Thomas splint, (A), when skeletal traction is used. When the pin-and-plaster unit is employed, (B), the calf of the leg is not compressed against the underlying slings by the weight of the limb.

that the moderator sling does not compress the soft parts behind the calf because these are suspended, free from pressure, by the Steinmann nail incorporated into the plaster (Fig. 141).

This detailed description of the traction unit may seem rather elaborate and even suggest that it is merely a gadget or a personal fad; I have used it, however, for several years and whenever I have abandoned it to try other methods I have usually regretted it and I have returned to the traction unit with the renewed conviction that it is a valuable appliance. Once the traction unit has been applied it can be left untouched for twelve weeks, making the maintenance of the case an easy nursing problem. During the 1939-45 war I found it possible to supervise thirty-five fractured femurs at one time with this traction unit, which would have been quite impossible using adhesive traction.

Suspension of the Splint

Using an overhead beam, the Thomas splint can now be suspended and counterpoised so that it moves easily when the patient moves in bed. If pressure of the ring against the groin is likely to be excessive, due to the amount of traction required, weight-traction can be applied to the foot of the splint which is added to the fixed traction already present (Fig. 142). Slight elevation of the foot of the bed will be necessary to counterbalance this sliding traction.

It will be noted that in this arrangement the addition of weight-traction does

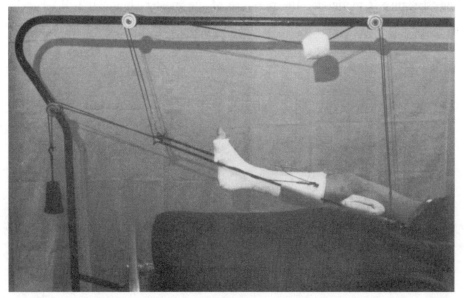

FIG. 142

Illustrating suspension of the Thomas splint, with pin-and-plaster traction unit, with the addition of a small amount of long-axis weight-traction to relieve pressure of the ring of the splint against the groin without seriously disturbing the attractive features of fixed skeletal traction. This makes the arrangement very comfortable for the patient.

not disturb the relationships between the site of the fracture, the splint, and the pressure pad, because the pressure pad is fixed to the splint and the fixed traction fixes the limb to the splint. In this way it is superior to many other methods where an increase in traction may cause the whole limb to move in relation to the splint and disturb the relationship between the pressure pad and the fracture. As long as the weight-traction is less than the fixed traction the full pressure of the ring against the patient will be alleviated and the mechanism of fixed traction will remain unaltered.

Comparison with the Braun Splint

Very few surgeons appreciate that there is any significant difference in the mechanics of this arrangement of the Thomas splint from the Braun splint which is so widely used on the Continent. While there is not much difference for a few minutes after the Braun frame has been adjusted the system of forces rapidly becomes ineffective, because the limb is able to move in relation to the splint. If the limb moves longitudinally in relation to the splint the site of the pressure pad will change in relation to the fracture. If the pelvis moves medially in relation to the splint, a varus deformity is produced because the knee is held by the splint. If the Braun splint had a ring to grip the top of the limb these defects would be eliminated ; but in that case it would be a Thomas splint !

Details of the Reduction

The reduction of an oblique, or comminuted, fracture is simple and can be carried out by the operator single-handed. The surgeon applies long-axis traction standing at the foot of the splint with one hand gripping the stirrup and applying

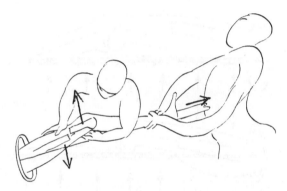

FIG. 143

Assistant and surgeon reducing a fracture of the lower
third of the femur.

counter-extension with the foot of the splint against his body to force the ring of the splint against the patient's perineum. The thigh is then laid on the pressure pad and the traction cords are tied to hold the position obtained by the initial powerful traction force.

If the fracture is transverse it will be necessary to have an assistant to exert powerful traction force while the operator concentrates on attempting to manipulate the fragments into apposition. With the assistant standing at the foot of the splint, exerting counter-pressure against it with his body and applying traction to the stirrup with both hands, the operator stands at one side of the splint and attempts to coax the fragments into alignment, testing for ' hitching ' of the bone ends by the ability of the fracture to resist telescoping when the traction is temporarily relaxed.

The commonest displacement is backward angulation of the lower fragment and the operator should therefore attempt to lift the lower fragment with his hand below the thigh, and press backwards the upper fragment with his hand in front of the thigh (Fig. 143). If resistance to telescoping is achieved the thigh is lowered on to the pressure pad, and the hand extracted from between the under surface of the thigh and the pad when the traction cords have been tied.

Radiographic control at this stage is of great value.

This manipulation is best carried out in the bed so that the final supervision of the splint can be performed without unnecessary disturbance.

A point of great importance concerns the displacement of the proximal fragment. It is inadvisable to apply a sling under the posterior surface of the thigh proximal

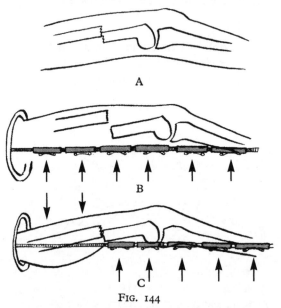

FIG. 144

Illustrating the danger of tightening the slings which underlie the proximal fragment. It is important to get a differential action by only supporting the leg, popliteal space, and the distal third of the femur, while the proximal fragment is allowed to fall backwards under its own weight.

A, Reduced position.

B, Displacement caused by tightening proximal slings.

C, Differential forces applied and reduction restored.

to the master sling. If this is done the proximal fragment is likely to be pushed forward and, although the fragments are still in parallel alignment, they will lose apposition (Fig. 144). In order to prevent this it is important to preserve a differential action of forces above and below the level of the fracture. Sometimes a reversed sling is useful at this point, *i.e.*, one passed between the side bars but in front of the proximal fragment to press it backwards.

Failure to Reduce a Transverse Fracture

Inability to secure the last $\frac{1}{16}$ inch of full length in a transverse fracture may mean all the difference between reduction and complete failure. Speaking generally,

I do not think transverse fractures of the shaft of the femur are suitable for conservative treatment; for these I advise the use of an intramedullary nail. If for special reasons it is necessary to treat a transverse fracture of the middle of the shaft of the femur conservatively and if simple long-axis traction fails to get full length, the method of increasing initial angulation may sometimes succeed. To do this the surgeon lifts the knee off the splint until the distal fragment is vertical and at right angles to the proximal fragment; he then pushes downward against

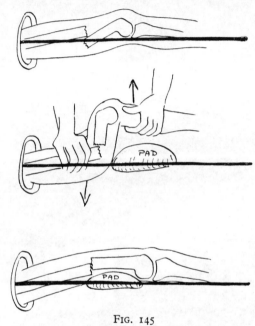

FIG. 145

Technique of reducing a transverse fracture in the lower third if longitudinal traction fails. Note that the master sling with its superimposed pad is applied to the splint *before* this manœuvre is executed because it is an important fulcrum in the actual manipulation.

the front surface of the proximal fragment while with the opposite hand maintain an upward pull on the distal fragment (Fig. 145). When the limb is straightened it can be deduced that the ends of the fragments are in contact if it is stable against a telescoping force.

When traction applied to a nail in the tibial tubercle fails to reduce an overriding transverse fracture, I have on occasions succeeded by changing to a supracondylar nail (Fig. 146). In the supracondylar region skeletal traction is more effective in its action on the distal fragment than equal force applied through the medium of the ligaments and capsule of the knee-joint when the tibial site is chosen for the nail. If supracondylar traction is used it should not be retained for more than two or three weeks, and the nail should thereafter be transferred to the tibial site. The ill-effects of supracondylar traction are the result of slight infection in the muscle planes which form the extensor mechanism of the knee-joint. Infection is inevitable if a supracondylar nail is left tco long *in situ* and if quadriceps exercises are attempted.

If a reduction is still not obtainable it will generally be found that the thigh is

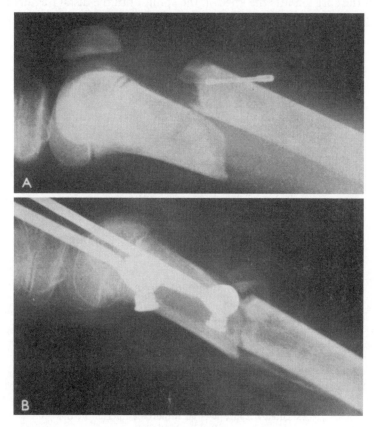

FIG. 146

Case of a transverse fracture of the shaft of the femur which resisted manipulative reduction using a tibial nail, but which was reduced by supracondylar traction.

grossly swollen and the barrier to obtaining full length is turgor from the effusion of blood into the closed fascial compartments of the thigh, which tend to assume a spherical shape, gaining in width at the expense of length. In this case, open reduction may be indicated after a delay of one or two weeks.

Abduction of the Splint

There is a constant tendency to the development of varus angulation in the conservative treatment of a fracture of the shaft of the femur. This is due to the powerful pull of the adductor muscles, and if any varus deformity starts these muscles are in an advantageous mechanical position to increase the deformity by a ' bow-string ' action.

A varus deformity is an unsightly deformity because it cannot be concealed in the standing position with the knees straight.

By maintaining the splint in considerable abduction throughout the post-operative course it is possible to counteract the action of the adductors and prevent a varus deformity (Fig. 147).

Watching the Ring of the Splint

In the post-operative course it is important to inspect the ring of the splint and the condition of the skin of the perineum in contact with it. By using 5 to 10 lb. of weight-traction the pressure of fixed traction against the skin can be mitigated, but it is important to make sure that the ring is not being pulled too far away from the perineum and lying in the region of the upper one-third of the thigh. This can only happen if the weight-traction severely exceeds the fixed traction inside the splint. If it is the result of slipping or stretching of the traction cords the ring can be approximated to the groin by shortening the fixed traction cords.

It is only by maintaining the ring close to the perineum that any control of the proximal fragment can be maintained. If the ring is allowed to take up a position in the middle of the thigh the method is no better than simple weight-traction applied to the distal fragment without any splint being used.

Post-operative Exercises

It is of fundamental importance to encourage the patient to try static quadriceps contractions as soon as he can after the apparatus has been set up. The patient does this by attempting to press the popliteal surface of his thigh against the pressure pad, at the same time endeavouring to lift his foot encased in plaster. Quadriceps contractions are encouraged by moving the knee as straight as possible, but control of the deformity of posterior angulation is best served by about 20 degrees of flexion of the knee.

In my experience the ability to perform quadriceps contractions early is invariably attended with rapid union and good callus formation in the radiograph at six weeks. It is impossible to say whether this is cause or effect; phlegmatic individuals seem to develop good callus, good quadriceps tone and early recovery of full knee motion, while the apprehensive patient is the reverse. Anything

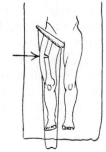

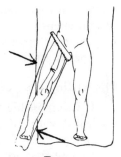

Fig. 147

Showing how the adducted position of the Thomas splint invokes lateral bowing and how the abducted position of the splint, which invokes medial bowing, anticipates this natural result of strong adductor tone. Note that in this illustration the fracture is in the midshaft of the femur ; this is not a suitable site for treatment by this method, unlike fractures in the lower third, and a Kuntscher nail is preferred by the author at this level.

which causes pain when an attempt is made to contract the quadriceps must be searched out and counteracted so that there is no reflex inhibition of muscle action.

After six weeks, clinical union may be developing so satisfactorily that it may be possible to change the system for simple skin traction. Skin traction at this stage is used merely to hold the Thomas splint in position so as to protect the fracture from angulation. When the skeletal traction is removed the Thomas splint should be changed to one with a smaller ring to adapt to the size of the thigh which by now will have lost considerable volume. At this stage the limb is splinted with the knee as straight as possible ; instead of the large pad producing 20 degrees of flexion which is necessary in the early stages, a small pad is used so that the knee is not flexed more than 5 degrees. This is important as it greatly facilitates quadriceps contractions. In this position it is possible for the patient now to acquire a longitudinal excursion of the patella of about ¾ inch in relation to the lower end of the femur. An excursion of ¾ inch of the patella is equivalent to about 40 degrees of movement in the knee joint, so that even if no movement of the joint is allowed the extensor apparatus can still be kept mobile in readiness for the time when the knee is set free.

Discarding the Splint

It is impossible to lay down any hard and fast rule for when splintage can be abolished with safety ; perhaps the following remarks will indicate the line of reasoning which I use as a guide. The danger at this stage is late angulation or even re-fracture. This is particularly the case in transverse fractures which have been reduced accurately end-to-end, because in these very little periosteal callus may be present and the mechanical strain on the callus is very great in a transverse fracture (see page 58). If knee stiffness is to be avoided some slight risk has to be taken, but if the following matters are appreciated, and if the surgeon supervises the matter himself, disaster should be avoided.

If the fracture is clinically firm by the first six to eight weeks the knee can be exercised, for short daily sessions, by the physiotherapist temporarily untying the traction cords and assisting the patient with straight-leg raising exercises and knee-bends. Often at this stage the patient is strong enough not only to elevate the leg but to elevate the splint and the leg in one piece. It is important, at this stage, that the cords are carefully retied at the end of each exercise with the splint ring well up in the groin. If the cords are carelessly tied and the groin ring is allowed to drift down the thigh, the ring will act as a fulcrum and instead of preventing will cause angulation.

The ultimate decision to abandon splintage entirely is often a little difficult. If the surgeon plays too much for safety there is a danger of prolonging the duration of knee stiffness more than necessary, while on the other hand he cannot toy lightly with the risk of re-fracture. It is dangerous to abandon the splint completely at three months if : (1) there is definite tenderness in the callus, (2) the amount of radiological callus is scanty or present only at one side of the fracture with none on the other, (3) there has been a constant tendency to late angulation which suggests defective consolidation.

Even if all these points appear adequate a re-fracture may still occur unless the surgeon is aware of *the significance of the range of knee movement in forecasting a threat of late angulation.* To make sure of this a record of gain in knee range

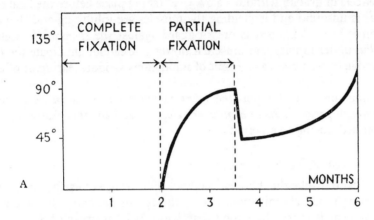

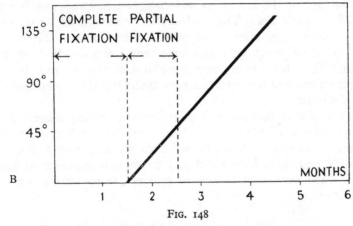

FIG. 148

A, Illustrating a sudden deterioration of knee movement after the thirteenth week, when all external support had been discarded. It is postulated that recovery was in abeyance until true consolidation of the fracture had been assured.

B, Illustrating a case in which strong bony union took place without incident and without any threat of re-fracture or late angulation. Knee movement returned spontaneously and progressively.

should be kept by the physiotherapist while intermittent knee exercise is being encouraged. When the decision is taken to try the patient out of the splint the patient should be allowed to sleep without the splint for one night, and the following day the range of movement in the knee joint should be measured. It will be found that the earliest sign of late angulation is a diminution of knee movement (Fig. 148). If the patient can get over a week without the splint and without losing the knee movement he had when the splint was abandoned he will have escaped the danger of spontaneous re-fracture or late angulation. This test depends on the fact that unsound callus is malleable and spontaneous fracture does not occur under the effects of gravity without a slow yield taking place before the final rupture. If the callus is unsound and is yielding the muscles are inhibiting and the range of knee motion is lost. This test is only a guard against the *spontaneous* yielding of *unsound callus* under gravity and muscular power ; it cannot anticipate the fracture of a thin bridge of true bone as a result of injudicious weight-bearing or of external strain.

Even using this test of union *the splint should rarely be abandoned completely before a minimum period of three months has elapsed*, and for this reason the patient must stay in bed during this period.

The Recovery of Knee Movement

For those who dislike the Thomas method, the absence of early knee movement appears to be the final abomination. Nevertheless, in the end result the recovery of knee movement is more often good than bad. It is surprising how knee movement will return spontaneously and continuously for as long as eighteen months following a fracture of the femur treated conservatively and this is particularly noticeable under middle age. The tendency to be pessimistic about any further recovery of the knee range after six months is often based on the bad prognosis of compound fractures which have had bone sepsis, and also because most other joints, especially the elbow, rarely gain more motion after six months. The stiff knee after a septic fracture is more intractable than after slow prolonged fixation in the absence of infection.

The recovery of knee movement is probably more closely related to biological matters in the process of bony union than to simple mechanical movement of the knee during treatment. A femur which is showing sound bony union by three months is certain to have rapid and continuous recovery of knee movement. Where knee movement is slow to recover the fracture almost invariably shows defective callus.

The Caliper Splint

In the original Thomas method the use of a caliper splint was a routine in the treatment of a fractured femur. The ' bed-splint ' was converted into a ' walking-splint ' at three months by cutting off the end of the splint and bending the ends to fit into holes drilled in the heel of a boot.

In the uncomplicated case a caliper is unnecessary. If clinical union has been present at eight weeks, it is quite certain that no caliper will be needed. If the fracture is a long oblique fracture there is certainly no need for a caliper (page 58). If the fracture is transverse greater caution is required, but even here, if clinical union has been present at eight weeks, if there is good callus at three months, and if the range of knee motion is improving progressively in the absence of splintage, there is no danger of re-fracture. If, however, callus is scanty, or restricted to one side only of the transverse fracture, and if the recovery of knee movement is slow or is stationary, the hazard of re-fracture must always be borne in mind, but even here a caliper splint is not always reliable in preventing re-fracture and in the modern world a prophylactic bone graft using the Phemister technique (see page 248) is advisable.

EXAMPLES:

In Fig. 149 are shown some of the results which are to be expected from this method. It is important to observe the standard of reduction which is to be regarded as praiseworthy; *half-diameters apposition in good alignment is to be regarded as perfect.*

Results

The only figures available for the results of treatment by the classical Thomas method (*i.e.*, three months in the bed-splint and three months in the caliper without knee movement) are those of Diggle (1944), and even these are only an impression of the results of 200 unselected cases; an average range of about 90 degrees was obtained after nine months with a maximum of $\frac{3}{4}$ inch of shortening. These results included the aged as well as the young.

In my own series of thirty-four cases (Charnley, 1947) only patients between the ages of twenty and forty-five years were studied, and only fractures in the middle and lower thirds of the shaft:

Average age . . . . . 26 years.
Start of knee movement . . . $10\frac{1}{4}$ weeks.
Average time of follow-up . . . 12 months.
Average final knee range . . . 128 degrees.

There were records of the knee range at six months in only twenty-seven of these cases; twenty-four of these had 90 degrees at six months = 88 per cent.

A comparable series which I selected from the published figures of the Massachusetts General Hospital (1930) (*i.e.*, twenty to forty-five years of age, closed fractures and middle and lower thirds) showed in eighteen cases:

Average age . . . . . 37 years.
Start of knee movement . . . 10 weeks.
Average time of follow-up . .. . . 15 months.
Average final knee range . . . 125 degrees.

In this series it is recorded that ten out of the eighteen had 'full' knee movement.

For the results of *early* knee movement in the treatment of this fracture Pearson (1918) used supracondylar ice-tongs and moved the knee at one month or as early as other factors allowed, and in sixty-eight cases there were fifty-five with 90 degrees at six months = 80 per cent.; Burns and Young (1944) in thirty-five cases with early knee movement on traction-suspension had thirty-one with 90 degrees at six months = 88 per cent.

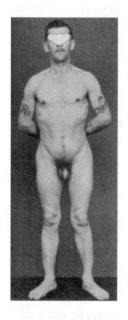
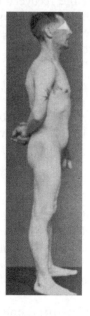

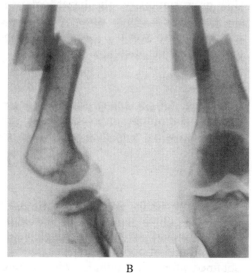

B
Right femur—before reduction.

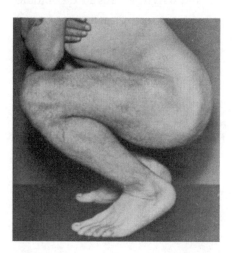

A

Bilateral femoral fractures; to maintain perfect alignment in both limbs throughout the treatment of a bilateral case is a rigorous test of the mechanical soundness of any conservative method; very slight valgus present in left leg.

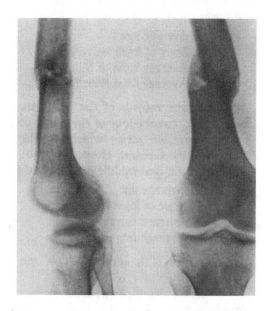

C
Right femur—united.

Fig. 149

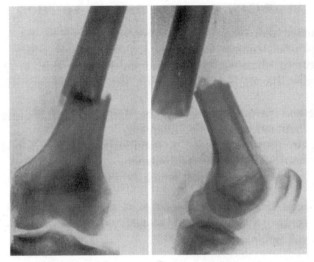

D

Left femur—before reduction.

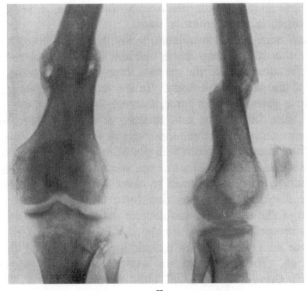

E

Left femur—united.

FIG. 149

SUMMARY OF THE THOMAS METHOD

1. It is claimed that, provided a manipulative reduction has been successful in getting end-to-end contact, this method is superior to operative methods of treating a fracture of the shaft of the femur in the *lower third of the femur*. The lower third, unlike the upper third, is not a site where internal fixation is easily applied.

2. This method permits traction to be decreased without prejudice to the stability of the alignment of the bone fragments.

3. The fracture must be reduced by manipulation. The method merely holds a reduction previously secured by manipulation.

4. Skeletal traction gives comfort which favours the start of active quadriceps contractions.

5. It is necessary to envisage three months in bed for the conservative treatment of a fractured femur : six weeks with skeletal traction and six weeks with skin traction and partial mobilisation.

Kirschner Wire versus Steinmann Nail

Many surgeons regard Kirschner wire and the Steinmann nail as alternative methods of applying skeletal traction ; that these are of equal merit, and that the choice of one or the other is largely a personal whim. The superiority of the Steinmann nail is so great, both in practice and theory, that it is important to state the reasons on which this contention is based.

The Kirschner wire moves in relation to the bone which it pierces ; the wire being solidly fixed to the stirrup which tightens it, every movement of the limb which changes the direction of the traction forces causes pivoting of the stirrup and movement of the wire in the bone. In the second place the pressure exerted on the bone, for a given traction force, is much higher with the Kirschner wire than with the 4 mm. Steinmann nail because of the difference in surface area. The Kirschner wire acts much in the same way as does the wire of a cheese cutter, but the 4 mm. Steinmann nail when well placed in thick cortical bone will remain firm for over six weeks. The Böhler stirrup, which is the best appliance by which to attach the traction cord, is designed to allow the stirrup to pivot freely on the nail even if the direction of the traction force changes through a considerable angle. By reason of the absolute immobility of the nail in the bone, sepsis is slow to start. Sepsis creeping inwards from the skin is abolished if the sealing of the punctures is done with an adequate technique. I have found that wool soaked in tinct. benz. co. (Friar's balsam) or Mastisol is highly satisfactory. Wool impregnated with these adhesives will cling as tenaciously to the steel of the nail as to the skin at the point of entry or emergence. This close adhesion to both skin and nail materially helps in checking movement between the skin and nail. Adhesives such as collodion on gauze do not 'bond' themselves to the metal of the nail, and thus movement can still take place between the nail and the skin and induce slight sepsis (Fig. 150).

In penetrating the skin with the Steinmann nail it is wise to incise the skin before inserting the nail or before allowing the point to emerge. This reduces the tension in the surrounding skin and minimises a slough. But more important than this is the careful inspection of the 'lie' of the skin around the points of

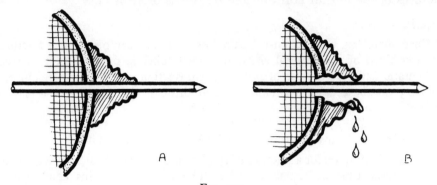

FIG. 150

Illustrating the importance of an adhesive.

A, Bonds to metal as tenaciously as to skin (*i.e.*, Mastisol or tinct. benz. co.).

B, Collodion will not bond to metal and movement is therefore possible between skin and nail, inviting ulceration and infection.

penetration to make sure that there is no pull in the skin to cause puckering of the skin on one side. This can be prevented by incising the skin on the puckered side (Fig. 151).

Sometimes a large ulcer can develop when a Steinmann nail is used without the piaster of the 'traction unit' (Fig. 141, p. 181). If the nail is inserted when the

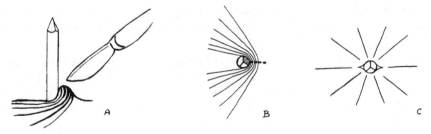

FIG. 151

The lie of the skin round the Steinmann nail; if the skin is puckered on one side a slough will result. This can be prevented by incising to equalise the tension.

calf muscles are dependent from the tibia, being unsupported from below, there is always a tendency for the skin to be pressed upwards against the nail when the leg is later made to lie on a splint. When the plaster of the traction unit is used, the soft parts of the calf are suspended inside the plaster and protected from pressure as the plaster lies on the splint.

These technical points in the use and upkeep of Steinmann nails are of great importance in their many applications to orthopædic surgery, and if they are observed there should be no difficulty in avoiding sepsis in nail tracks for as long as three months.

Fractures of the Femur complicated by Burns or Skin Loss

Os Calcis Traction

When there has been extensive skin loss or burns complicating a fracture of the lower third of the femoral shaft, the tibial tubercle may be unfit to receive a Steinmann nail, and the use of skin adhesive traction may similarly be out of the question; in these cases a Steinmann nail through the os calcis may save the situation.

Fractures of the Femur complicated by Fracture of the Tibia

It is not uncommon for a fracture of the femur to be complicated by a compound fracture of the tibia on the same side. The treatment of this combination is discussed on page 243.

Fractures of the Shaft of the Femur in Children

Up to about ten years of age the treatment of fractures of the femoral shaft should be dictated by principles of the utmost simplicity. It is almost unnecessary to use radiological control because the external appearance of the limb is the essential thing.

During the first three weeks after the injury the surgeon should concentrate on the length of the limb while maintaining alignment only very approximately. Any form of adhesive traction may be used (*i.e.*, fixed Thomas after five years of age, Bryant's suspension under five). During this initial three weeks a shortening of $\frac{1}{2}$ inch should be considered ideal. Full length is not advisable as there is a danger of growth being stimulated by the fracture and of the final length of the leg being excessive.

After three weeks callus will be present and no recurrence of shortening will result if traction is removed. Traction can therefore be removed and a single-sided hip-spica should be applied, under anæsthesia, so that a careful moulding of the plastic callus can be obtained. The plastic callus can be bent like bending a lead pipe and we avoid the problem of controlling angulation in two planes simultaneously, as is necessary in a fresh fracture. Using radiological control at this stage an accurate correction of alignment can be obtained and easily held.

Using this technique of planned 'delayed moulding' (*cf.*, fractures of radius and ulna in children, page 124) the treatment of these fractures is not only very simple but it is also rendered very precise.

REFERENCES

BURNS, B. H., & YOUNG, R. F. (1944). *Lancet*, **1**, 723.
CHARNLEY, J. (1947). *J. Bone Jt Surg.* **29**, 679.
DIGGLE, W. S. (1944). *Lancet*, **2**, 355.

CHAPTER FOURTEEN

FRACTURES OF THE FEMORAL AND TIBIAL CONDYLES

T HE injuries specially to be considered under this heading are : (1) T-shaped supracondylar fractures of the femur, (2) fractures of the medial femoral condyle, (3) T-shaped fractures of the tibial plateau, and (4) depressed fractures of the lateral tibial condyle.

The principles which should dominate treatment must take into account the following three features :

1. They are fractures involving a joint.
2. They are fractures of cancellous bone and are either comminuted or impacted.
3. They occur commonly in elderly patients and only rarely in athletic age groups.

These features demand a method with the following requirements:

1. Early mobilisation because the joint is involved.
2. Avoidance of traction and the encouragement of ' controlled collapse.' Controlled collapse in fractures of cancellous bone favours rapid consolidation and therefore indirectly promotes the return of joint mobility.
3. Acceptance of radiological deformity if clinical deformity is not gross. This is often made possible by the patient's age and is part of the principle of ' controlled collapse.'

When these principles are observed the rate of consolidation and recovery of joint mobility in elderly patients is sometimes quite astonishing. It is no uncommon thing to find a fracture quite painless at three weeks under this regime. In the patient, aged eighty-one, illustrated in Fig. 152, the T-shaped supracondylar fracture of the lower end of the femur was treated on a Thomas splint with fixed traction. While permitting collapse of the fracture from its original position after reduction the shortening became excessive (Fig. 153). Because I was worried lest the projection of the sharp spike of diaphysis would impede movement of the extensor apparatus, I attempted a remanipulation ; but even after only two *weeks* the fracture could not be moved under full anæsthesia. Twelve weeks after fracture this patient had 90 degrees of knee movement and was walking without pain, though at that time she could not actively extend the last 10 degrees. The final result was excellent.

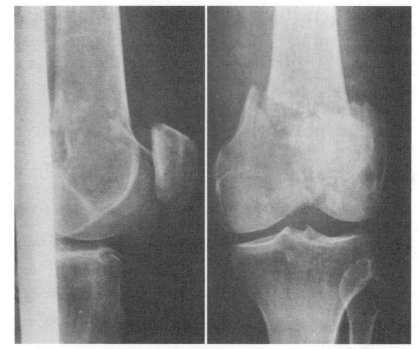

FIG. 152

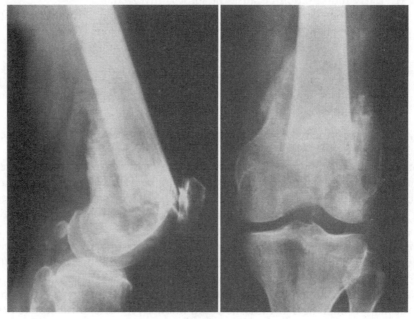

FIG. 153

Weight-Traction and Early Knee Mobilisation

Excellent functional and anatomical results have been obtained in fractures involving the knee joint by weight-traction and early movement without splintage (Fairbank, 1954; Apley, 1956). I have no wish to decry the use of weight-traction without splintage in fractures involving the knee joint, and it is possible that I may be over-exaggerating the dangers of breaking down impacted fractures in cancellous bone by the use of weight-traction; nevertheless I still think that, *as a principle*, one must secure the start of sound consolidation before attempting joint movement if to procure joint movement introduces factors capable of impeding consolidation. The example illustrated in Fig. 154 is that of a frail woman, sixty-five years of age, treated with ' controlled collapse ' on a Thomas splint with fixed traction. Movement inside the bandages was encouraged from the beginning, intermittent release of the knee was started at the end of three weeks, and all splintage was discarded at five weeks; 90 degrees of flexion was obtained at the end of seven weeks, and eventually a practically normal knee resulted. This speed of recovery of function and of knee range could not have been exceeded by any weight-traction method with early joint movement.

A disadvantage of the Thomas splint method is that it requires the daily attendance of a physiotherapist to untie and re-tie the traction cords. On the other hand, the method has a very important advantage over the skeletal traction in that control of alignment in the extended portion of the knee is possible and there is no danger of the infection of a fracture hæmatoma at the upper end of the tibia by a Steinmann nail applied in the area of tissue involved in œdema and ecchymosis.

An interesting example of conservative treatment in a fracture of the lateral femoral condyle is illustrated in Fig. 155 which occurred in a vigorous male of forty-five years of age. It is probable that many surgeons would have applied a transverse screw. Treated on a Thomas splint in the manner described the tendency to valgus deformity was minimised and intermittent mobilisation was started after three weeks. Function was so good that all splintage was abandoned after five weeks and the patient went home on crutches with 90 degrees of knee range. The end result was indistinguishable from normal and therefore the result of arthrotomy and internal fixation could not have been better. The only justification for operating on this fracture would have been a post-operative radiograph with a ' hair-line ' reduction, and to get this might require a much more extensive arthrotomy than the operator expected at the start of the operation; to end the operation with an imperfect reduction would merely be meddlesome interference. If an attempt had been made to insert a screw it would have had to be inserted proximally in order to keep clear of the sliding mechanism of the joint capsule (a feature which does not complicate the insertion of screws transversely across fractures in the head of the tibia).

Technique

The mechanical principles involved in the treatment of all fractures involving the knee joint by means of the Thomas splint are the same whether the fracture is in the condyles of the femur or the tibia. The position of the fracture is

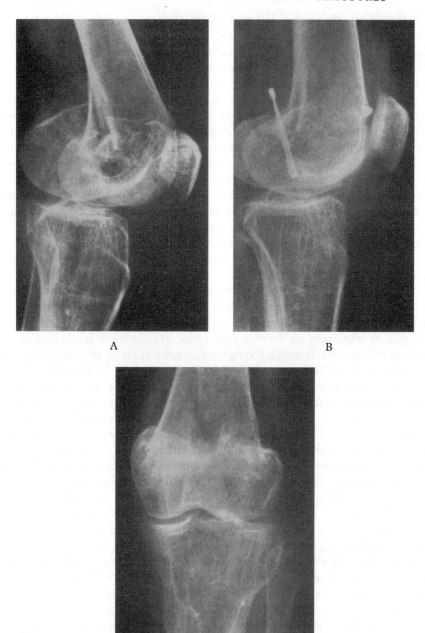

A   B

C

FIG. 154

Supracondylar fracture of femur in lady of sixty-five, treated by 'controlled collapse,'
on straight Thomas splint, with skin extension for five weeks. Note knee range of
90 degrees seven weeks after injury.

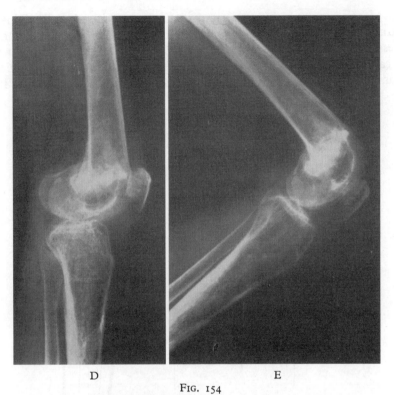

D   E

FIG. 154

Supracondylar fracture of femur in lady of sixty-five, treated by 'controlled collapse,' on straight Thomas splint, with skin extension for five weeks. Note knee range of 90 degrees seven weeks after injury.

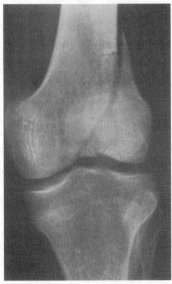

FIG. 155—Fracture of lateral femoral condyle in man, forty-five years of age. Treated conservatively in preference to use of a transverse screw (see text).

FIG. 155

'improved' (it is a euphemism to say that the fracture is reduced). This is done by getting an assistant to apply a traction force while the surgeon manually compresses the affected part of the knee from side to side, or from front to back, as the case may indicate. This is done after skin traction has been applied and a Thomas splint is in place. With the knee resting on the Thomas splint it is now

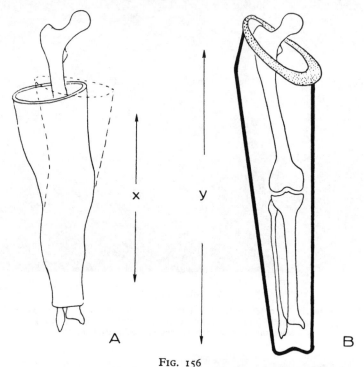

FIG. 156

Illustrating mechanical inefficiency of a plaster groin-ankle cylinder, A, in controlling angular deformity at the level of the knee, when compared with the long levers available in a Thomas splint, B. Short length of control (x); long length of control (y).

possible to control the amount of shortening by the skin traction and at the same time to correct the valgus deformity.

Very few people appreciate the mechanical advantage of the Thomas splint with fixed skin traction for injuries such as this in comparison with a plaster cast. It is necessary to emphasise that the Thomas splint permits an accurate control of valgus deformity because it takes a fixed purchase in the groin; in this respect it is superior to the inefficient control exerted by a plaster cylinder on a thick, short, and flabby thigh (Fig. 156). It is probable that those who fail to appreciate the mechanical advantage of the Thomas splint do so because they do not have the authentic apparatus with its complete ring and do not possess a suitable range of sizes; often what is called a 'Thomas splint' is nothing more than a variety of first-aid appliances with a ring which is so large that it can be applied outside the trousers, or which has a half-ring wrapped only in wool and a cotton bandage.

The Thomas splint is better than a plaster cylinder because *it allows* the *surgeon to observe the rate of clinical union* by detecting the earliest indications of the return of function. If a plaster cylinder is used it has to be applied for an empirical time of four to six weeks, but on a Thomas splint the sign that the knee is ready to start some active movement between two and three weeks after the injury will be evident when the patient is able to lift the knee a short distance off the pad lying under it. This movement is done with the heel still resting on the splint and is possible long before the patient can do a ' straight-leg raise.' The knee is not ready for the start of active joint movement until the patient can actively lift it a short distance inside the bandages holding it to the splint. There is no apparatus, except a Thomas splint with *fixed* traction, which simultaneously permits (1) incomplete immobilisation, (2) the control of varus and valgus angulation, and (3) the limb to be maintained with a controlled amount of shortening. It might be argued that simple balanced traction with weights and pulleys would facilitate knee movement and control angulation in a more comfortable and convenient way than the Thomas splint with fixed traction. But weight-traction can only control angulation when the intermuscular fibrous septa are pulled taut and this means that the limb is pulled out to full length. No other apparatus exists other than the Thomas splint with fixed traction, which allows the limb to remain slightly short (controlled collapse) without at the same time interfering with the efficiency of the mechanism controlling alignment.

It will be evident from this account how little the radiological control helps in the treatment of these cases. The recovery of motion in a joint where articular surfaces are involved by a fracture is quite unrelated to the amount of displacement; trivial displacements can often result in very stiff joints.

Résumé of Technique

To show the basic simplicity of the method the stages in treatment can be re-stated thus :

1. Under general anæsthesia apply skin traction to the leg, thread a Thomas splint over the thigh, and attach slings between the side bars to support the region of the knee.

2. With an assistant applying longitudinal traction to the foot, compress the knee from side to side and lower the limb on to the slings of the splint.

3. Attach the traction cords to the foot of the splint.

4. With tape measure or X-ray control, allow the limb to shorten a trifle after ' improving ' the position.

5. Encourage quadriceps contraction and watch for the first sign of the patient being able to lift the knee an inch or so off the splint—this will be about three weeks after the injury. By this I mean lift the knee with the heel still on the splint ; it will not, of course, be possible to execute a ' straight-leg raise ' until much later.

6. When signs of active knee lifting are seen, untie traction cords daily and get a physiotherapist to support the limb and encourage active flexion exercises.

7. Abandon the splint when active straight-leg raising is easy (four to eight weeks) and rest knee on a pillow.

8. Do not worry if a little valgus deformity recurs in elderly patients—it will not be seen under a long skirt or in trousers.

9. Permit weight-bearing between eight and twelve weeks.

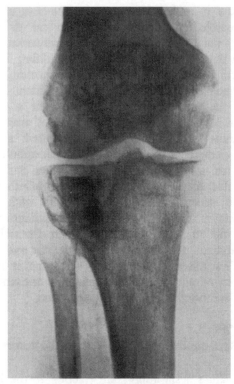

FIG. 157

Showing the result of open reduction in a depressed fracture of the tibial plateau—ischæmic necrosis of the fragment after operative elevation. Late traumatic arthritis likely though immediate result may be good.

Indications for Operative Treatment

Operative treatment is indicated in the relatively uncommon cases encountered in persons of athletic age, and especially where the fragments appear to be held apart by a down-driven fragment separating them. In these cases it is necessary to perform a complete arthrotomy and usually to remove a cartilage to expose the tibial plateau in order to raise the depressed fragment to the correct level (Fig. 157). In these younger patients a transverse screw is probably the best way of approximating the separated fragments.

REFERENCES

APLEY, A. G. (1956). *J. Bone Jt Surg.*, **38B**, 699.
FAIRBANK, J. T. (1954). *Proc. R. Soc. Med.*, **48**, 95.

CHAPTER FIFTEEN

FRACTURES OF THE SHAFT OF THE TIBIA

THE bad results of open reduction and internal fixation of fractures are most commonly seen in fractures of the shaft of the tibia. There are several reasons for this : the tibia is the commonest major long bone to be fractured; it is very commonly a compound fracture ; it is a fracture which is easily exposed and therefore tempts inexperienced operators ; it is a subcutaneous fracture and after plating is especially prone to defective wound healing accompanied by what in some quarters is euphemistically termed ' drainage.'

We have still a long way to go before the best method of treating a fracture of the shaft of the tibia can be stated with finality. I feel sure that a closed method will eventually prevail, but we need mechanical aids to improve our control of the bone fragments. It is possible time will show that an intramedullary rod, introduced through the tibial tubercle, *without exposing the fracture site*, will be enough to enhance alignment as an adjuvant to closed methods. Used in this simple way the intramedullary rod will not be responsible for immobilisation ; it will merely control alignment and prevent slipping of the reduced fracture.

Most surgeons who practise internal fixation of tibial fractures do so with the idea that accurate coaptation of the fragments, combined with rigid fixation, enhances the ability of the fracture to unite. I have attempted to show in Chapter I that this mechanical approach to fracture healing is out of touch with biological reality.

When viewing the excellent results which are often demonstrated as attributable to the plating of fractures of the tibia we must never forget that the best results of operative treatment are in cases which would also give excellent results by simple plaster fixation. In other words, rapid osseous union after plating the fractured tibia is not a result of the plating but a result of factors resident in the soft tissues associated with that particular fracture.

Example.—Fig. 158 illustrates what might have been shown as an excellent example of the advantages of operative treatment of a fractured tibia. The criticism I wish to make is that the good result should not be credited to the operation. The deformity in the initial radiograph is little more than simple angulation which could have been corrected by manipulation. The anteroposterior radiograph shows that the original deformity was convex at the attachment of the interosseous membrane where an intact periosteal bridge could therefore be predicted. *This prediction is confirmed by the final radiograph which shows plentiful callus at the tibial attachment of the interosseous membrane.* The essential feature which this case illustrates is not the efficacy of internal fixation *per se* but merely that internal fixation has here been used on a case highly favourable for normal osseous union under conservative treatment; it does not indicate that a similar gratifying result would be obtained in a case with gross stripping of all soft tissue attachments as a result of severe initial displacement with overriding of the fragments.

In considering the bad results of plating of fractures of the tibia it is not an exaggeration to say that amputation after one or two years of disability from a fracture of the tibia, can almost always be traced to an injudicious plating operation at the time of the original injury. No fractured tibia, no matter how extensively comminuted, necessitates early amputation by reason of the magnitude of the shattering or loss of bone; early amputation is invariably a sequel to serious damage to major blood vessels and nerves, to gas gangrene, or to extensive loss

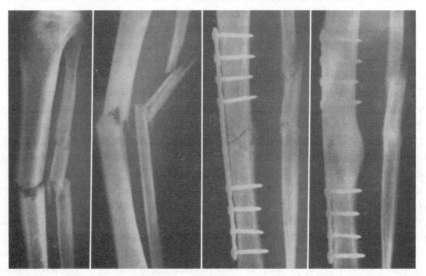

FIG. 158

Successful result of internal fixation but not to be used as a general argument for internal fixation in tibial fractures. Original displacement suggests soft tissue callus pathway probably intact (Group A, Fig. 160, page 210). Union by simple conservative method could be predicted. Note callus bridge at attachment of the interosseous membrane.

of skin. If a patient with extensive comminution of a compound fracture of the tibia survives these initial hazards, osteomyelitis which may follow under conservative treatment is never so profound as to require amputation. Sequestra involving a complete segment of the tibial diaphysis are never encountered after the conservative treatment of the most extensively compound comminuted fractures. The tubular sequestrum in traumatic surgery is invariably the result of infection superimposed on operative interference. Infection demarcates in a permanent fashion the volume of bone rendered ischæmic by the procedure of applying a plate and six screws.

To condemn the plating of fractures of the shaft of the tibia as a maxim in the teaching of safe surgical methods, must not be taken as a total condemnation of this technique. Many exponents of this method can show an impressive series of results, but I believe that this is not so much the result of the method as the result of finely developed clinical perception in the pre-operative selection of cases and in the awareness of threatened post-operative complications for which appropriate avoiding action is promptly taken. In the hands of the unwary this method can lead to disastrous results as indicated in the following example which was perpetrated by a general surgeon who was a competent operator.

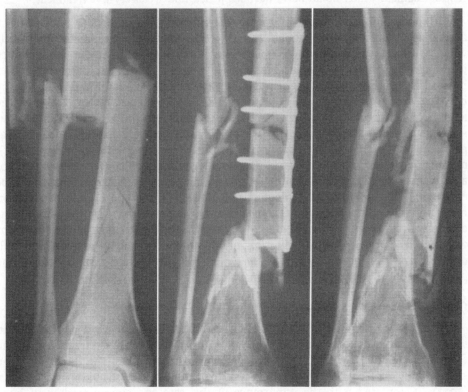

FIG. 159

Bad result from internal fixation. Tubular aseptic sequestrum (see text).

Example.—Fig. 159. This example illustrates a disaster of the first magnitude which could not have occurred after conservative treatment. The operator underestimated the significance of the undisplaced crack in the distal fragment; he embarked on what he thought would be a simple plating operation on the main fracture. During the operation the undisplaced crack separated completely, and because the fracture lay too near the ankle a second plate could not be applied. The attempt to insert an oblique screw was futile and the operator, wisely in the circumstances, decided to close the wound with the deliberate intention of applying a cancellous bone graft after two or three months. Unfortunately, when the wound was reopened three months later for the grafting operation it was found that the whole of the middle fragment was completely ischæmic. It was so ischæmic that when the plate was removed the proximal end had not even united to the proximal fragment of the tibia though the fracture had been completely immobilised, and had not had any leverage exerted on it. The application of cancellous bone grafts to distal and proximal fractures was not successful and the illustration shows radiological evidence of ischæmia of this tubular fragment. There was never any infection in this case. It is possible that on economic grounds this patient eventually may have to submit to below knee amputation, because even after two years, and after a second cancellous bone graft, there is still no union. Plating this fracture precipitated total ischæmia of the central fragment which would never have happened under conservative treatment.

In condemning the primary operative treatment of fractures of the tibia the crucial argument concerns the evil effects of the open exposure of the fragments which is seen at its worst when a plate is applied to the tibia under the mistaken idea that rigid fixation encourages osseous union. There are, however, other methods of improving the precision of conservative treatment which lie half way between conservative principles and operative. It is possible to stabilise the alignment of fractures of the tibia by the use of an intramedullary nail, even without seeking to produce rigid internal fixation. Intramedullary fixation such as that proposed by Rush can be performed without exposing the fracture or with minimal exposure of the fracture. Used as an adjunct to conservative treatment as a method of giving some precision to the maintenance of alignment, this type of fixation does not offend biological principles. This type of internal fixation need not aspire to rendering external fixation unnecessary. In the subsequent discussion the only form of operative treatment I shall encourage in the treatment of tibial fractures is the stabilisation of alignment by the intramedullary nail, inserted *without exposure of the fracture*, and not demanding a rigid hold of the point of the nail in the distal fragment.

Conservative Treatment and the Phemister Bone Graft

The greatest advance in the treatment of fractures of the shaft of the tibia in the last half century has not been in techniques for the primary treatment of the fresh fracture, but has been in the secondary management of the fracture by the simple sub-periosteal bone graft which was first put on a scientific basis by Phemister (1947). Compared with the importance of this safe and simple method of bone grafting (which I shall describe in detail later) the relative merits of conservative and operative treatment of the initial fracture are almost insignificant.

I will justify this sweeping statement by reference to two special features of the Phemister graft using strips of autogenous iliac bone. Firstly, the resistance to infection shown by this graft and its ability to succeed even in the presence of mild infection are such that it becomes possible to use a bone graft very much earlier than was considered possible in the past. Secondly, the flexibility of the individual strips of cancellous bone renders it possible to apply a graft in the presence of mal-aligned fragments. To use a cortical bone graft, either onlay or inlay, in these circumstances would be courting disaster.

Using the Phemister type of bone graft three months after the injury it becomes possible practically to guarantee osseous union, with all external splintage finally abolished, six months after the most severe fracture of the tibia. According to the strategy of using the Phemister graft at three months no attempt is made to adopt radical operative measures for initial treatment in the hope of getting primary union in three months. A more consistent level of success over a large series of cases will be achieved by planning conservatively at the beginning, but being radical in employing a Phemister bone graft as soon as this is first indicated at about three months.

According to these tactics the fractured tibia is treated during the first two or three months with attention devoted primarily to giving time for the revascularisation of the fragments and the avoidance of procedures likely to increase the volume of ischæmic bone already resulting from disruption of the longitudinal circulation in the ends of the fragments. The initial period of delay gives time for the skin and soft parts to recover from the immediate effects of trauma. This emphasis on the nutrition of the soft parts is not only applicable to compound fractures; it is too commonly forgotten that the skin overlying a closed fracture of the tibia is treacherous material through which to operate. The difficulty in wound closure after primary operative treatment of the tibial fractures frequently leads to defective wound healing. Skin which is prone to develop fracture blisters, as is the skin over the subcutaneous border of the tibia, is obviously far removed from normal, and in this respect the tibia is much less suitable for open exposure than are bones which are well covered with muscle. It is sometimes argued that this early involvement of skin in a fractured tibia makes it imperative that open reduction should be performed as early as possible after the injury and before the skin has had time to become œdematous; this recommendation pays no attention to the inevitable behaviour of the skin some days after the wound has been closed and lost from sight under the dressings.

Selection of Type of Treatment

By considering the nature and magnitude of the displacement of the tibial fragments it is possible to select the most appropriate form of treatment for the individual case. The initial radiograph may help in estimating the magnitude of displacement, but most important of all is the clinical examination of the limb with the patient under anæsthesia. It is possible for the initial radiograph to underestimate the magnitude of tearing of the soft parts as a result of the fracture being roughly aligned in the course of first-aid work.

From this assessment two predictions can be made: (1) from the stability of the fracture it can be decided whether it is suitable for the simplest of conservative methods or whether the stability will require to be enhanced by an intramedullary nail, and (2) a prediction can be made regarding the likelihood of delayed union. If from the magnitude of the displacement it is predicted that delayed union is likely to be encountered, strategy must be planned to render the limb in perfect condition for bone grafting should mobility still be present at ten or twelve weeks.

The reader must not get the impression from this account that I am suggesting that almost all tibiæ should have a Phemister graft at three months. The decision to perform the graft is made on the presence or absence of clinical

INITIAL DISPLACEMENT MODERATE

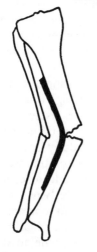

NO REDUCTION NEEDED
or
CORRECTION OF ANGULATION
ALONE REQUIRED

Intact Periosteal Hinge, Minimal
Disruption of Interosseous Membrane

| 1 | 2 | 3 | 4 |

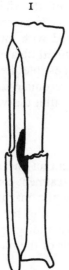 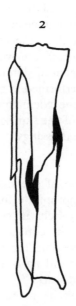 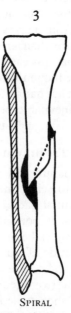 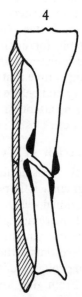

TRANSVERSE	OBLIQUE	SPIRAL	OBLIQUE WITH GAP
		Fibula intact (or undisplaced)	*Fibula intact* (or undisplaced)

SIMPLE PLASTER FIXTURE ADEQUATE   DELAYED UNION POSSIBLE
(Intramedullary rod may
be advisable)

A

Fig. 160

INITIAL DISPLACEMENT SEVERE

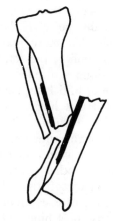

REDUCTION IMPERATIVE—SIMPLE CORRECTION
OF ANGULATION NOT ENOUGH

Periosteal Hinge and Interosseous Membrane
completely disrupted.   Shortening present

Delayed Union very likely
Bone graft to be considered at three months

RADIOGRAPHIC APPEARANCES AFTER MANIPULATIVE REDUCTION

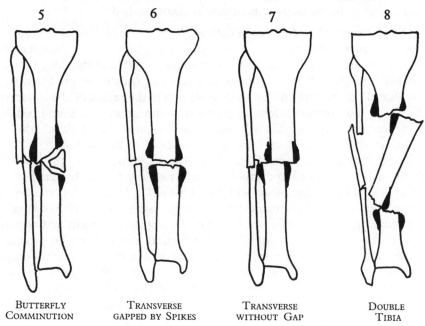

5	6	7	8
BUTTERFLY COMMINUTION	TRANSVERSE GAPPED BY SPIKES	TRANSVERSE WITHOUT GAP	DOUBLE TIBIA

McKEE METHOD or
Stabilise with Intramedullary rod as adjuvant to plaster.

AVOID OPERATION
(Graft end which is still
mobile after three months)

B

FIG. 160

211

union at three months and the majority of fractured tibiæ do not require a bone graft. In the past the commonest error in treatment has been the too long postponement of bone grafting. If postponed too long the condition of *pseudarthrosis* may be established and this condition is more difficult to graft than is a simple case of delayed union. Early bone grafting according to this policy is therefore a form of 'prophylactic grafting.' Though it is possible that more grafts are performed than are absolutely necessary according to this policy, the total time of disability over a large series of several fractured tibiæ will be reduced.

In assessing the original fracture as regards the degree of initial displacement, the essential feature is to decide whether an ' intact soft-tissue hinge ' is likely to be present because this favours union by conservative methods. The soft parts most vitally concerned in conducting osseous union across the tibial fragments lie in the interosseous membrane where that structure is attached to the tibia. Callus is seen at this point even when it is absent at other parts of the tibial fracture. It is to be noted that I am using the term ' intact soft-tissue hinge ' both in a biological sense, as a pathway capable of conducting osseous union from one fragment to another, as well as in the mechanical sense of a hinge whereby the displaced fragments can be guided into position during manipulative reduction.

Two grades of initial displacement can be distinguished :

1. Displacement nil, or little more than angulation. *In all these cases the fracture can be put into an acceptable position simply by correcting angulation.* Such shortening as there is can be accepted because the fracture is stable at this length and will not shorten further. An intact soft-tissue hinge can usually be predicted on the concave side of the fracture and this will usually be in the region of the interosseous membrane. Union usually offers no problem in this group and sound consolidation under conservative methods will usually be present within three months. The types of cases encountered in this group are indicated in Fig. 160, A.

2. Displacement with overriding. Here the attachments to the interosseous membrane will be ruptured and this important pathway for the bridging of callus from one fragment to the other will be destroyed. Delayed union even after accurate coaptation of the fragments will be likely. Simple correction of angulation is not enough in this type of fracture. The restoration of length and apposition by at least half diameters is essential. Mechanical means must be provided to render the reduced position stable. According to the biological ideas proposed in this work the method required to render the fracture stable against redisplacement need not provide rigid fixation. The types of cases encountered in this group are indicated in Fig. 160, B.

In this second group of fractures of the tibia and fibula the need to prevent redisplacement after reduction is particularly important if the limb is encased in a plaster cast. If a fracture of the tibia and fibula has been reduced by applying traction and a plaster cast, there will be a grave risk of ' plugging ' of the venous return inside the plaster if the fracture redisplaces when the traction is removed. Traction lengthens the leg, at the same time making it narrow, and when traction is released the limb will increase in thickness inside the plaster at the same time as it shortens. The vicious circle of venous obstruction which can result from this type of 'plugging' is exceedingly dangerous and especially so if the after-care of these cases has to be entrusted to relatively inexperienced residents during the vital twenty-four hours after reduction. Attempts to assess the circulation by pressing on a toe, to observe the return of blood into the blanched area, are notoriously unreliable and have often given reassurance that the circulation was intact when reassurance was not warranted. It should be emphasised that severe post-operative pain must not be regarded as a normal sequel after the satisfactory reduction and fixation of a fractured tibia. Any patient who is not rendered comfortable by a single dose of morphia after reduction of his fracture may have a serious vascular complication, and this must be diagnosed during the first six or twelve hours after the application of the plaster. The loss of sensation in the toes, and especially loss of active movement of the toes, are both serious signs even in the presence of what may seem to be a good circulation as judged by pressure of the finger on the nail-bed.

Transverse Fractures of the Tibia

The management of transverse fractures of the tibia showing gross initial displacement is a difficult problem. Even if excellent end-to-end reduction is achieved by closed manipulation, the chances of delayed union are still great because this has been decided by the magnitude of the initial displacement. Internal fixation will not enhance the power of union. There is a serious risk of redisplacement if simple plaster fixation is used when the initial displacement has been gross. For this reason it is advisable to consider stabilising the alignment of such a fracture by an intramedullary nail.

Example.—Fig. 161 illustrates this point. The patient was sixty years of age and delayed union was predictable as a result of the magnitude of the original displacement. Predictable also was, or ought to have been, the possibility of redisplacement by treating such a fracture in a simple closed plaster without any additional mechanical assistance. This case should have been supplemented by an intramedullary nail used to stabilise alignment rather than to provide rigid fixation. The patient should be warned as soon as possible after the original injury that an early bone graft will probably be performed in view of the magnitude of the original displacement. If on examining the state of union three months after this injury it is evident that osseous union is present or in progress, the patient will be delighted to learn that no bone graft will be necessary, but if free mobility is present the patient is already adjusted to the idea and the news does not come as a shock.

In treating transverse fractures of the tibia with gross initial displacement the surgeon should be particularly warned of the possibility of delayed union when full diameters apposition has been obtained by closed reduction. I suggest that sometimes an inexperienced surgeon may be so pleased to see full diameter apposition achieved as a result of his closed manipulation that he may overlook the fact that the fracture has been 'gapped open' by spikes which, like the teeth of a gear wheel, may not be completely in register. The bone spikes which gap the fracture open are almost certain to be totally ischaemic. When apposition is only

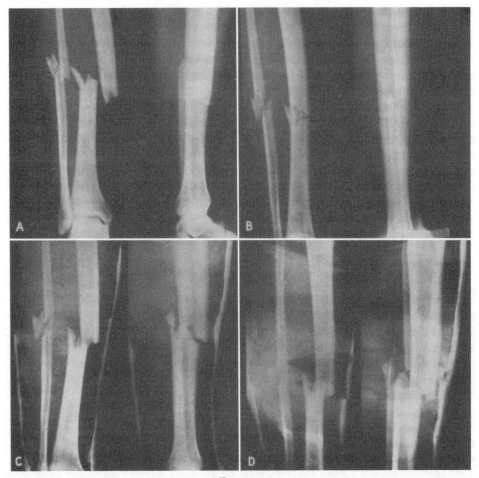

FIG. 161
Example (see text).

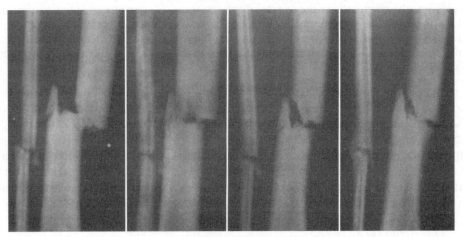

FIG. 162
Example of the gapping open of a transverse fracture by a spike (see text).

by half diameters it is more likely that the fragments will have sunk towards each other more completely.

Example.—Fig. 162. This patient was a man of forty-five years of age with a closed transverse fracture of the tibia and fibula. After manipulative reduction the transverse fracture is seen strutted apart by an unlucky position of the projecting bone spikes. Measured direct on the X-ray film there is a gap of 4 mm. between the bone ends. Eight weeks later there is not the slightest evidence of bridging of the gap which is now reduced to 3 mm. on the X-ray film. Close inspection of the periosteal surfaces of the fragments indicates early periosteal activity and the fibular fracture is already showing good callus. Sixteen weeks after the injury the fracture was still completely mobile. The gap between the bones was now diminished to 1 mm. as the result of weight-bearing in plaster.

This patient was submitted to a bone graft six months after the injury. From the original displacement and the presence of mobility at three months, this patient ought to have had a Phemister graft at three months rather than this should have been delayed to six months.

According to the biological principles advocated in this work open reduction of this fracture with accurate coaptation of these bone spikes would not have enhanced the power of osseous union.

The correct strategy in this case would have been to plan treatment with a view to grafting early because the surgeon could have been forewarned by examining under anaesthesia the magnitude of displacement of the original fracture.

In considering the role of intramedullary fixation in a case such as the foregoing, it must be emphasised that the absence of rigid internal fixation is not a disadvantage in this technique. If osseous union is not in the process of development three months after the injury it is better for this to be revealed by clinical examination of the fracture than to have it masked by the internal fixation which may render the tibia 'plate-solid' and delay the diagnosis of defective consolidation until failure splint of the internal brings this to light at a much later date.

The Butterfly or Wedge-shaped Fragment

One of the most treacherous tibial fractures which may invite the unwary surgeon to operate is that in which one main fragment is roughly transverse and the other is oblique, as the result of the separation of a wedge-shaped (butterfly) fragment. The danger in this fracture lies in the fact that the wedge-shaped fragment cannot take an active part in union, because its longitudinal Haversian circulation must be seriously interrupted, and operative intervention will render it even more completely ischæmic. If in our mental image we exclude the butter-fly fragment from the active process of union, we see that after reduction the main tibial fragments are in contact only at one small point, at the summit of two spikes, and that the greater part of the fracture is a 'gap' bridged only by the metallic fixation (Fig. 163). The two main fragments demand that they be approximated towards each other and, if possible, that one spike should fit inside the medullary canal of the other. Moreover, being a comminuted fracture it is devoid of the potential stability which is produced by the interlocking of non-comminuted fractures in the reduced position, and the metallic splint used for the internal fixation of this type of fracture will be directly exposed to all the deforming forces without any protection or reinforcement from the bones themselves (as can happen to some extent in transverse fractures), and it is likely that failure of the fixation will occur.

The conservative treatment in this type of case can be reinforced by an intra-

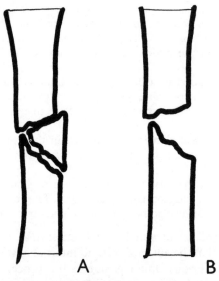

FIG. 163

Diagram to illustrate idea that ' butter-fly ' fragment, A, plays only passive role in osseous union (especially if devitalised by open operation). Bio-logical state of such a fracture is as if fragment was absent, B.

medullary nail to hold alignment provided that this is inserted without exposing the fracture site.

Oblique Fractures of the Tibia with Intact Fibula

When this type of fracture is first seen it often seems so innocent that it is frequently put into a plaster cast without anæsthesia. Reduction is often considered unnecessary because the displacement appears so slight ; and an anæsthetic is not needed during application of the cast because the intact fibula offers splintage. This fracture is a frequent source of delayed union and is the solitary exception to the general rule that delayed union is most frequent after gross initial deformity.

The strutting action of the intact fibula causes the tibial fragments to 'float' near each other so that they frequently separate in a lateral direction. If several films are taken with the leg in different degrees of rotation a clear gap may be

216

demonstrated between the tibial fragments (Figs. 164 and 165). This gap is accentuated by the tendency for the tibia to angulate towards the intact fibula. These remarks apply with almost equal force when the fibula is fractured but undisplaced.

Delayed union in this type of fracture is often quoted against the argument that the magnitude of the initial displacement governs the speed of union. It is

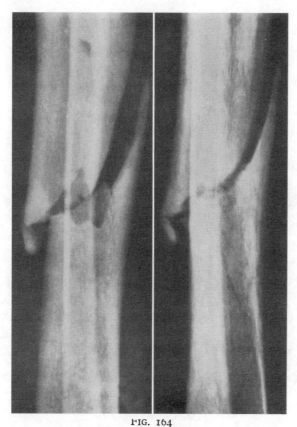

FIG. 164

Example of fracture with gap held open by an intact
fibula which proceeded to delayed union.

probable that the flexibility of the fibula, and the flexibility of the upper and lower tibio-fibular joints, masks the fact that at the moment of injury this tibial fracture might have been grossly displaced with extensive separation of the fragments from the interosseous membrane, and disruption therefore of the natural pathway for callus.

Oblique fractures are unsuitable for fixation by a transverse screw. The fragments have to be denuded fairly completely in order to obtain a ' hair-line' fit of the fragments, and the strength of the fixation is poor in resisting movement in the plane of the fracture.

Spiral Fractures

It is necessary to emphasise that *spiral* fractures of the tibia, even if associated with an intact fibula, almost never show non-union. If a fracture is truly spiral it will be impossible (by definition) for a clear gap to be seen through the fracture by any orientation of the radiograph. The displacement of a true spiral fracture, especially if there is a trace of shortening, produces some degree of interlocking

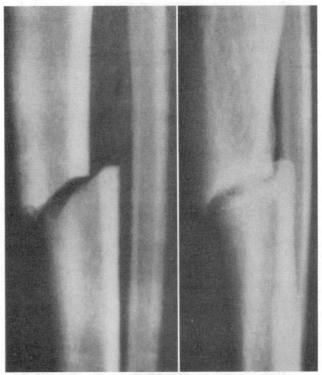

FIG. 165

Example of fracture with gap held open by an intact fibula which proceeded to non-union.

of the fragments, with ideal contact of periosteal and endosteal surfaces, and there is never much tendency for a spiral fracture to angulate towards the fibula and so to open a clear gap by lateral displacement.

The Unreliability of the Transverse Screw

It is often tempting to coapt the fragments of an oblique or spiral fracture of the tibia by one or two transverse screws transfixing the fragments. Though at one time a keen exponent of this method, I am now reluctantly forced to advise caution in its use and to recommend that only one screw should be used (for coaptation not fixation), periosteum should be disturbed as little as possible, and plaster fixation should be used thereafter as for closed treatment. The depression of biological activity in a healing fracture as a result of operative exposure of the fracture has been mentioned in Chapter I (pp. 21-27), and the mechanical strength of this method of fixation is not enough to withstand the strain over the prolonged period of time to which it is exposed as a result of the artificially delayed process of union (Fig. 26, p. 25).

An example of the harmful effect of three screws traversing the bone ends actually involved in a fracture is seen in Fig. 166. At operation, undertaken because the fracture was completely mobile four months later, the bone ends were visibly ischæmic for a distance of nearly 1 cm. on each side of the fracture.

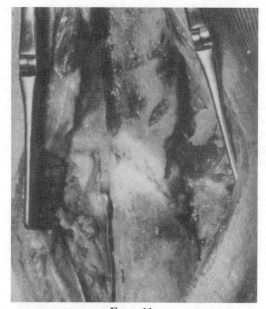

FIG. 166
Un-united fracture of the tibia, short oblique, four months after insertion of three transverse screws. Note dead white bone ends adjacent to the line of the fracture.

The insertion of screws and the stripping of periosteum accentuates a state of affairs already existing to some degree after any fracture of a long bone.

It is not commonly realised that the use of *two* screws across an *oblique* fracture does not produce such sound mechanical fixation as *one* screw on a *spiral* fracture. When a *spiral* fracture has been accurately coapted it becomes locked under light pressure and thereafter can resist quite powerful stresses in a variety of directions. The total strength of this junction is largely due to the locking of the spiral bone fragments and the screw is shielded from most of the external forces exerted on the tibia. The *oblique* fracture, however, unlike the spiral fracture, occupies only a single plane, and therefore it has no locking potential and has no inherent stability against motion in that plane. The truth of this statement can easily be tested experimentally. Oblique fractures therefore expose the screws to extreme strains because the fixation is entirely dependent on the strength of the screws. There is evidence also that two or three transverse screws can devitalise the oblique fragment if separated by less than about 1 cm. from each other, and thus increased mechanical fixation may have the disastrous effect of causing widespread bone death.

It is an ironical fact that it is the oblique fracture of the tibia which most often invites operative coaptation (when in combination with an intact fibula), whereas the spiral fracture of the tibia, which is mechanically suitable for a transverse screw, never needs to be operated on because it never presents a gap.

Only too often a fracture which is regarded as a simple spiral at operation will be found to be comminuted as a result of a minute crack which was not detected in the original radiograph. It is foolish to persist with attempts to insert several transverse screws in these cases.

It should be unnecessary to remind the reader that if a transverse screw is to be applied to one of these fractures the screw hole in the superficial cortex (*i.e.*, that which will eventually be in contact with the head of the screw) should be larger than the outside diameter of the screw thread, and that only the deep cortex, which receives the point of the screw, should be drilled to 'tapping size.' Failure to observe this technical point is a common source of trouble, but I have seen failures in the treatment of oblique fractures with a transverse screw even when this detail has been carefully observed (as in the case illustrated in Fig. 26, p. 25).

Double Fractures of the Tibia

The 'double' fracture of the tibia, in which there is a large central fragment comprising practically the whole of the middle third, should never be treated by open operation (Fig. 167, A). The danger of converting the whole of the central fragment into a dead tubular sequestrum by operative interference is too great to be worth the risk. It is worth emphasising that large pieces of the tibia which can be seen to be dead when exposed during bone-grafting operations do not reveal themselves by increased density on the radiograph (Compere, 1949).

The safest way of handling these double fractures is by conservative treatment followed three months later by a planned bone graft (predicted to the patient). The leg can be kept at adequate length (*i.e.*, encouraging a little shortening) in a simple plaster cast without traction. After three months one end of the large central fragment (usually proximal) will be clinically united while the other end will be mobile. A graft of iliac bone (p. 248) can now be applied to the un-united fracture and a further three months of plaster fixation will see the successful conclusion of a very difficult problem in a total period of disability of no more than six to nine months. It is unnecessary to consider the position of the central fragment, because the alignment of proximal and distal fragments in relation to their associated joints is easily controlled, and if gross deformity is accepted the opportunity can be taken at the time of bone grafting to reduce the size of any ugly bony prominence by shaving it away. The serious danger of prolonged invalidism —and even amputation—which can follow injudicious handling of this very difficult fracture cannot be over-emphasised. An example of this fracture treated

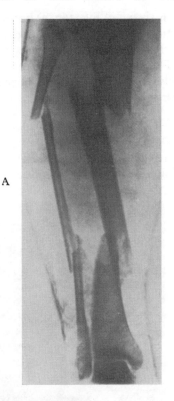
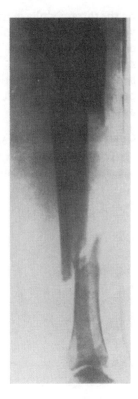

A

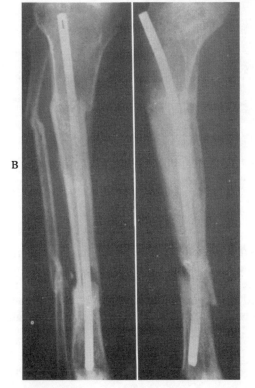

B

FIG. 167

Double fracture of tibia. Internal fixation gave good radiological result, B, but fixation had to be reinforced by plaster and the distal fracture developed non-union. It would have been better to have used the conservative method and accept the original deformity (see text).

by the intramedullary nail is shown in Fig. 167, B; but after a very difficult operation, where the threat of infection as a result of prolonged handling of the tissues was only avoided by good luck, non-union still developed in the distal fracture and needed bone grafting. The patient was therefore no better off than if he had been treated conservatively from the start, and it was necessary to use a plaster because the intramedullary nail did not completely immobilise the fragments against rotation.

Cosmetic Factors in Conservative Treatment

It is sometimes forgotten that the final appearance of a leg after a fracture of the shafts of the tibia and fibula can usually be judged from the external appearance

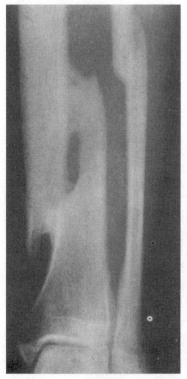

FIG. 168

Extreme example of deformity not suspected by external inspection of leg. Patient was a heavily built man. Union first detected six weeks after fracture.

of the limb when the plaster is about to be applied. The stark simplicity of this recommendation can be appreciated when one realises that this approach is almost a return to the methods of the Middle Ages. A gross example, which I do not suggest should be copied, is illustrated in Fig 168; this degree of displacement would never have been suspected by external inspection of the leg one year later and this carries with it an important lesson. There is a danger in being satisfied by the radiograph, as a criterion of parallel alignment, if the surgeon does not take care also to *look at the shape of the leg with his naked eyes*. This paradox is encountered if the surgeon is about to accept the position of a fracture where the proximal fragment is lying, as it most often does, more medial than the distal fragment (Fig. 169). If the distal fragment is aligned in strict radiological parallelism with the proximal fragment a visible

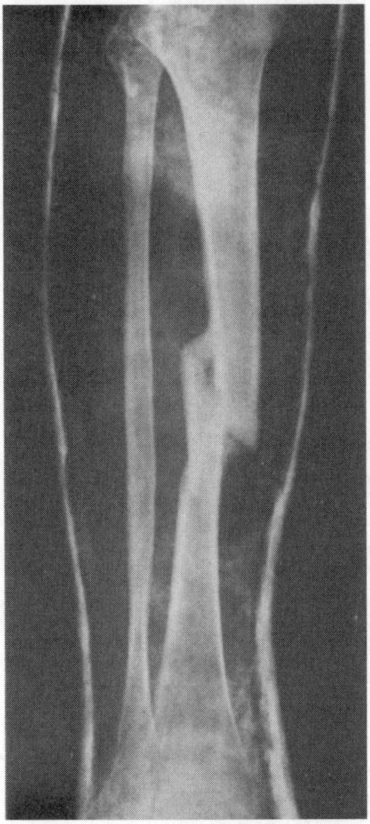

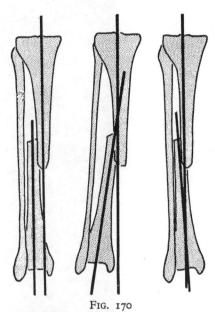

Fig. 169

Bony prominence on subcutaneous surface of tibia, caused by proximal fragment, is made cosmetically more objectionable by slight valgus deformity of distal fragment.

Fig. 170

Showing how classical advice to align tibial fragments in exact parallelism is neither cosmetically nor physiologically sound if the fragments have some lateral displacement. Valgus deformity is always cosmetically objectionable; but a trace of varus deformity will conceal a bony prominence and bring centre of ankle joint back into line of weight-bearing.

prominence may be caused on the subcutaneous border of the tibia. A slight valgus deformity in such a case will make this prominence even more ugly. On the other hand, and this is the point I wish to emphasise, a slight varus deformity, deliberately introduced by the surgeon, will conceal such a bony boss (Fig. 170). Other examples of this are indicated in Figs. 171 and 172. The amount of varus required is nothing more than is needed to bring the centre of the ankle joint back into the line of the axis of the proximal fragment. Insistence on strict radiological parallelism will place the centre of the ankle joint lateral to the natural axis of weight-bearing.

223

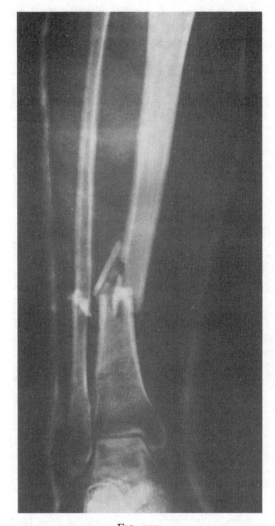

FIG. 171

Excessive *varus* angulation yet external deformity
was not particularly noticeable. Axis of proximal
fragment in line with tibiofibular joint, whereas it
should lie near centre of talus.

The statement which one routinely hears that an angulation as small as 5 degrees
will inevitably cause late traumatic arthritis of the ankle joint is not supported
by the facts. I cannot recall an example after a fracture involving only the shaft
of the tibia, though it is of course common when the ankle joint itself has been
directly involved in a fracture.

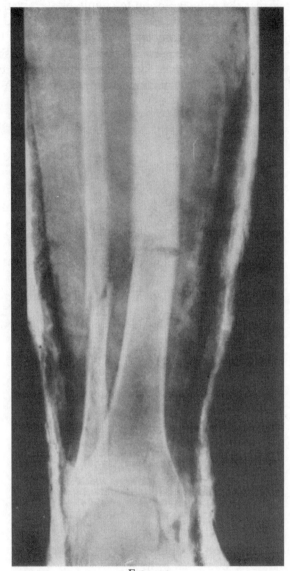

FIG. 172

This trivial amount of *valgus* angulation was cosmetically objectionable, because it destroyed the concave profile of the subcutaneous surface of the tibia.

TECHNIQUE OF CONSERVATIVE TREATMENT

1. Simple Plaster Fixation

The fractures of the tibia chosen for this type of treatment will be judged from the magnitude of the original displacement and will fall into the categories shown diagrammatically in Fig. 160, A.

225

It is to be noted that the only exception to simple plaster fixation in this group of relatively undisplaced fractures is the oblique fracture of the tibia associated with the intact fibula. I suggest that this type of case should be submitted to intramedullary nailing if the displacement is severe. This point should be judged under general anæsthesia rather than from simple inspection of X-ray which may minimise the problem. If on testing under anæsthesia the fracture is not

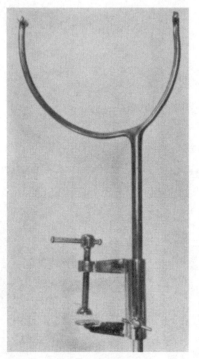

FIG. 173

Simple support for knee which can be attached to any table. Bandage is passed across the open end of the U which is then placed behind the knee.

unstable and is no worse than would seem to be apparent from the X-ray, it is probably unnecessary to use internal fixation.

Having decided from the original displacement that the stability of a fracture against further shortening renders it suitable for simple plaster fixation, to hold a manual reduction while applying a long leg plaster in one stage is a very difficult matter. I have found the following technique better than the alternative of applying first a below-knee plaster, with the knee flexed, and later completing the plaster above the knee.

It is essential to have a fixed support for the knee rather than to expect an assistant to hold it manually. The device which I have adapted from the Putti orthopædic table (Figs. 173, 174, A, B, C) has proved useful. The knee is supported on a flannel bandage tied across the free ends of the support and, in order to extract it easily when the plaster has set, it is liberally covered in a tube of wool which is left behind in the plaster.

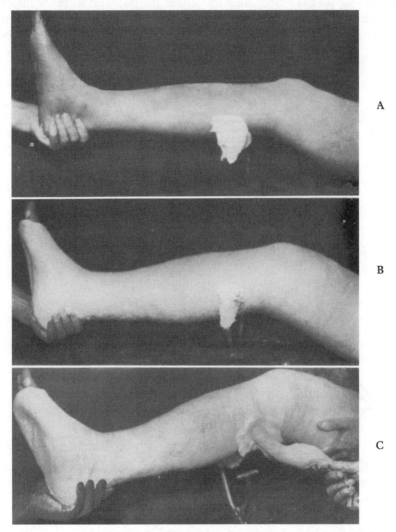

FIG. 174

Use of knee support.

A, Wool-covered support in position.
B, Plaster applied.
C, Support being extracted after being cut.

It must be emphasised that there is a very serious danger of obstructing the popliteal vessels by this support if the operator does not understand the method of extracting it as soon as the plaster has hardened. The tubular covering of wool is applied to prevent the flannel bandage adhering to the plaster and remaining inside the cast as a constricting ridge.

A technical detail is illustrated in Fig. 175 : it will sometimes be found that if the knee support is placed directly behind the popliteal fossa the upper fragment will sag into posterior angulation (Fig. 175, A) ; to overcome this the knee support should be placed behind the upper quarter of the tibia.   In order to encourage the

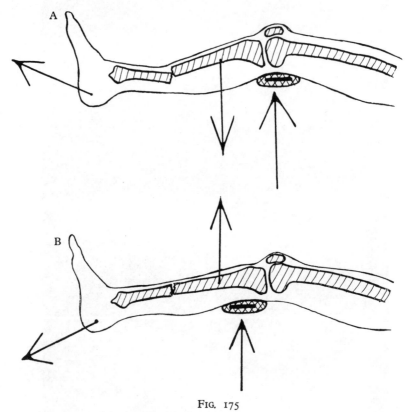

FIG. 175

Diagram explaining necessity, in some cases, for supporting tibia behind upper quarter rather than behind the knee joint, to hold forward proximal fragment and prevent backward angulation.

normal tendency to a concave curvature on the subcutaneous border of the tibia, the best position for the leg is rolled outwards in slight external rotation (Figs. 174, C, and 176).

The plaster should be padded with an even layer of wool ½ inch thick, placed over stockinet, and the plaster bandages applied with firm tension to compress the wool and enhance fixation.

At this initial stage under anæsthesia the foot should be brought up to the right angle, though an exact plantigrade position should not be too much of a fetish if thereby posterior displacement of the fracture is invoked.   If the foot cannot

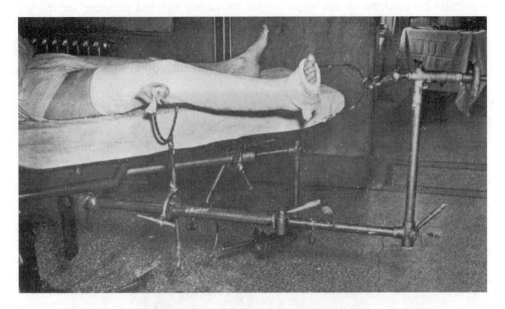

229

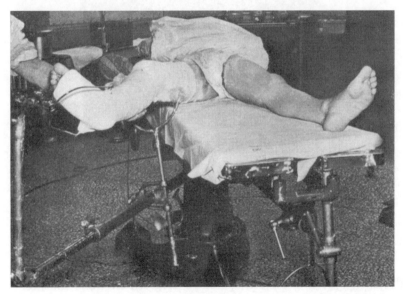

FIG. 176

Alternative arrangement using temporary skeletal traction on the heel. Note the external rotation which converts undesirable tendency to backward angulation into desirable position of varus bowing.

easily be brought up to the right angles by gentle upward pressure on the sole of the forefoot, this must be combined with manual traction to the heel; this combination of traction on the heel and upward pressure on the forefoot is better than powerful forcing of the forefoot dorsally, which tends to cause backward angulation of the fracture. The best stance for the surgeon is with the sole of the

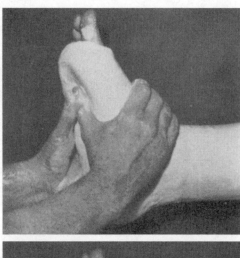

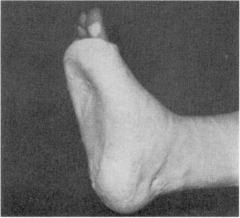

FIG. 177

Moulding sole of plaster to restore transverse
metatarsal arch.

patient's forefoot resting on the operator's epigastrium while the heel is pulled down with one hand.

If, when the plaster is complete, the foot should be in some equinus, I strongly recommend that when the plaster is to be changed at six weeks, in preparation for walking, it should be done *under full anæsthesia*, because without anæsthesia it is never possible to bring the foot to the right angle no matter how the patient tries to co-operate.

The transverse metatarsal arch should be moulded into the sole of the plaster as the last stage after the main body has set (Fig. 177).

Wedging the Plaster

The judicious use of intramedullary nailing in difficult fractures of the tibia will reduce the necessity for wedging of plasters, but there will always be a place

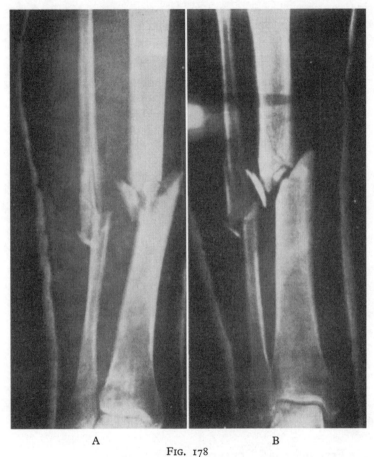

A   B

FIG. 178

Wedging plaster by *opening concave* side can distract and displace a fracture.
This case developed non-union, as might have been predicted from the gap.

for this procedure which should be regarded as an unfortunate necessity rather than a procedure of choice. If the radiograph shows some residual angulation, this can be corrected by wedging.

The common and easy method of wedging a plaster, by cutting it on the side to be made convex and strutting open the saw cut with blocks of wood, may have deleterious effects by distracting the tibial fragments (Fig. 178). I have the impression that the tibiæ which present with delayed union show an unusually high proportion which have been wedged in the course of their early treatment.

The truth of the matter is that cases such as that illustrated in Fig. 178 proceed to delayed union as a result of the magnitude of the initial displacement rather than as a result of the wedging.

The best method of wedging is to close the plaster on the side to be made concave. There is here a danger that the skin may be pinched in the gap if a narrow wedge is removed, and it is much better therefore to cut a large window in the convex side so large that it is still widely open when the wedging has been completed. The plaster can then be completed without pinching the soft parts (Fig. 179).

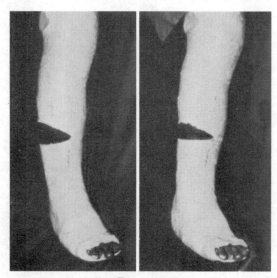

FIG. 179

Wedging plaster by *closing convex* side of deformity.
Necessary to remove a wide wedge so that it is not
completely closed at the end of wedging and so cannot
pinch soft tissues.

All wedging should be finished within the first two or three days after reduction, and the first plaster should then be left untouched for six to eight weeks.

2. Unstable Fractures and Conservative Treatment

The fractures in this category are shown diagrammatically in Fig. 160, B. *The tactics in handling this type of fracture are to avoid major primary operations and concentrate on the possibility of an early Phemister bone graft if mobility is detected three months after the injury.*

These fractures are unsuitable for simple plaster fixation, as after reduction and traction the possibility of slipping is very great.

These cases can be treated by skeletal traction according to McKee's method outlined on page 235. By this technique the alignment is held for four to six weeks and a plaster cast then applied when shrinking of the soft parts has become maximal, and when redisplacement of the fragments is unlikely. Six weeks later the plaster is removed and the condition of union estimated clinically with a view to proceeding immediately with a Phemister bone graft.

Intramedullary Stabilisation

In this category of unstable fracture with gross initial displacement the idea of an intramedullary nail of the Rush type is very attractive if it can be inserted *without opening the fracture*.

After insertion of the nail the fracture is managed as for conservative methods in a long-leg plaster for three months and the condition of union at the end of this time is assessed with a view to immediate Phemister bone grafting without further delay. In inserting the intramedullary nail it is important to have strong skeletal traction to align the fragments by a screw traction device such as the Watson-Jones screw tractor which is used with the knee flexed to 90 degrees over the edge of the table.

Compound Fractures of the Tibia

In the common type of compound fractures of the tibia, where a small wound is present as a result of the bone penetrating the skin from within, the treatment is identical with that for a closed fracture if the skin is clean and no more than about six hours have elapsed since the injury.

When a compound comminuted fracture of the tibia and fibula is complicated by extensive loss of soft parts and skin, the problem is much more difficult. The treatment of this type of injury by a simple plaster technique is unsatisfactory because some infection is unavoidable and venous obstruction due to ' plugging ' of the leg inside a plaster cast, in the absence of traction, can have a disastrous effect on the healing of slightly infected wounds.

It has been argued that the immobilisation of bone fragments is more essential in an open fracture than in a closed fracture, because if the fragments are allowed to continue in free mobility it is possible that bacterial contamination may proliferate and a more extensive infection occur than if the fragments were not in relative motion. With this object in mind there are some surgeons who apply plates and screws to compound fractures of the tibia, especially with skin loss, because the internal fixation facilitates an immediate cross-leg skin graft to obtain bone cover. It is argued that if infection should occur it will be nothing more serious than a mild local infection around the plate, which eventually subsides when union at a later date permits the plate to be removed. Remarkable successes have certainly been recorded by this technique since the advent of antibiotics, but we must not forget the cases where operative intervention in these circumstances has been the deciding factor in precipitating complete ischæmia of full-diameter sections of the tibial graft, necessitating amputation one or two years later after prolonged disability. I have already mentioned that late amputation as a result of osteomyelitis does not happen when a fracture has been treated conservatively at the outset.

It is possible that there may be a revival of interest in external skeletal fixation in a restricted field of application to compound fractures of the tibia necessitating skin cover. In this technique the proximal and distal fragments are transfixed, through healthy skin and at some distance from the fracture, by 'half-pin units' which are then connected together by a rigid external steel bar as in the Stader splint (Fig. 180). Unfortunately when this method was practised in the U.S.A. and Canada during the Second World War it was grossly abused and is now in disrepute. Nevertheless the principle of this method offers the best theoretical conditions for an open fracture of the tibia to heal without bone infection. External skeletal fixation should be restricted exclusively to the treatment of fractures of the tibia and fibula and should not be used for any other bone. The bad reputation which this splint has acquired is the result of its abuse. The transfixion pins should never penetrate muscle, because the movement of muscle round the nails, which occurs if associated joints are exercised, will induce infection. The patient should never be expected to become ambulant with external skeletal fixation *in situ*. The patient should not be allowed to hold the limb dependent and engorged

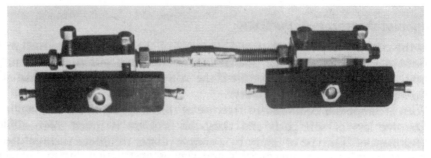

FIG. 180
Stader splint. See text.

with blood for long periods of time. The external skeletal fixation should be removed as soon as the condition of the compound fracture permits and should not be retained *in situ* for months in the hope of union occurring.

In a series of animal experiments undertaken to compare the rate of union after different forms of mechanical fixation, Hey Groves (1921) came to the conclusion that external skeletal fixation gave the best callus formation of any method he had tried. In this comparison he used plates of various sizes with different forms of attachment, such as screws and 'split-pins,' and also intramedullary fixation. To quote Hey Groves :

'There can be no doubt, as far as the evidence of these experiments goes, that this method of indirect fixation of the fracture gives a more perfect union of the bones than any direct method that I have performed.'

Skeletal Traction

A popular method of handling severe fractures of the tibia and fibula is to apply skeletal traction to the lower end of the tibia or os calcis, and nurse the limb on a Braun splint. Usually the alignment of the limb is reinforced by the application of a below-knee plaster.

This method lacks precision in that the proximal fragment is not controlled, and if there has been extensive damage to soft parts, weight-traction of 10 lb. may produce considerable distraction of the fragments. If it is considered necessary to reinforce the fixation with a below-knee plaster, this has the disadvantage of rendering the wound inaccessible. The method of external skeletal fixation which I have found best (McKee's method) uses a bent Thomas splint to replace the Braun splint, and the proximal fragment is held to the splint by means of a second nail. In this method fixed traction is used so that the length of the tibia can be set at whatever length the surgeon wishes.

In this method it is unnecessary to use plaster and the leg is supported with flannel slings and the wound can be dressed and skin grafted by Thiersch or pinch grafts at any time in the subsequent course of healing.

I consider this method is preferable to the simple technique of incorporating transfixion nails in plaster. A single Steinmann nail in the proximal and in the distal fragments in combination with a plaster cast is not enough to control angulation in two planes, but in combination with a Thomas splint there are facilities for readjusting the alignment in stages subsequent to the original reduction.

By concentrating on procedures to obtain skin closure, while holding the fracture in acceptable position, it is almost always possible to get the soft parts healed and dry and in a state suitable for grafting by the Phemister technique in the most severe of compound fractures of the tibia before three months have elapsed.

The compound tibia is held with skeletal fixation on the splint with the patient in bed for an initial period of four to six weeks, and thereafter a long leg plaster is applied and the nails are removed.

Details of Technique. McKee's Method.

A new Thomas splint is chosen with a ring of suitable diameter to fit the opposite groin. The splint is bent 30 degrees at the point which will correspond with the level of the knee. This is easily done by bending over the edge of a table.

The patient is anæsthetised and the skin cleansed with soap and water, etc., prior to surgical debridement of the wound. Having surgically cleansed the wound, the leg can be draped in sterile towels while the Thomas splint is threaded over the limb and while the Steinmann nails are being inserted. It is unnecessary to insist on very strict asepsis during this phase of the procedure as the nails can be inserted by no-touch technique. The side bars of the Thomas splint can be sterilised by antiseptic means such as wiping down with a suitable antiseptic solution.

The first Steinmann nail is inserted into the proximal fragment at the level of the tibial tubercle and every care should be taken to see that this is transverse to the long axis of the proximal fragment.

The second Steinmann nail is now passed through the os calcis. This must be done below the side bars of the splint with an assistant holding the splint upwards.

The proximal Steinmann nail is now clamped to the side bars of the splint using the McKee clamps (Fig. 181) in a position which brings the ring of the splint in comfortable relationship with the groin.

McKee clamps are now threaded over the distal nail which is loosely clamped to the side bars *underneath* the splint (Fig. 182).

Powerful traction is applied to the distal nail with the surgeon standing so that the foot of the splint is against his body (Fig. 183). The distal McKee clamps are now tightened and the position of the fracture under powerful traction is assessed. At this point the splint can be draped with sterile towels and the fracture and wounds exposed. Direct inspection of the fragments can be carried out, and the effect of reducing the traction from the distal nail can be examined. The object is to find the minimum amount of traction which will hold the fragments in stable alignment.

In the case of closed fractures radiographic control will help in the final adjustment of the reduction.

When the position of the fracture is regarded as satisfactory, dressings are applied to the wound and flannel slings placed under the calf to check posterior sagging.

It is finally necessary to support the forefoot to prevent a cavus deformity taking place at the midtarsal joint. This can be done by means of a plaster slab which can be bandaged to the side bars of the splint with a figure-of-eight bandage.

Post-operative Management

The patient can be nursed in bed with a rigid support to hold the heel clear of the bed (Fig. 192, B, p. 243) or preferably the splint can be counterpoised from a Balkan beam (Fig. 192, C, p. 243).

After three or four weeks there may be considerable shrinkage in volume of the soft parts, especially if the leg originally was grossly swollen with effused blood. It may be necessary to re-tighten the slings if shrinkage of the leg has permitted posterior bowing to occur.

Throughout the four weeks X-ray checks should be made from time to time with a view to readjusting the first alignment of the fracture if necessary, and for this purpose short anæsthetics may be needed.

Application of the Final Cast

After four to six weeks the fracture will be sufficiently sticky to permit it being held in a long leg cast without the transfixion nails. This can be done without anæsthesia by applying wet plaster slabs to the front and back of the leg and thigh and bandaging into position with gauze bandages while the limb is still held in the splint. When these plaster slabs have hardened the splint can be removed and the slabs converted into a complete cast after removing the splint.

Special Details

Two special details in the handling of severe compound fractures of the tibia by this method need emphasis : (1) Landmarks for inserting the nail in the os calcis. It is important to avoid transfixing the subastragaloid joint with the distal

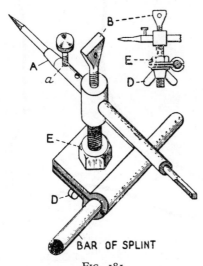

FIG. 181

McKee clamp for holding Steinmann
nail to the side bars of the Thomas
splint.

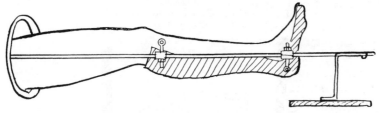

FIG. 182

McKee clamps on Thomas splint with plaster slab to reinforce fixation against
movement in a sagittal plane.

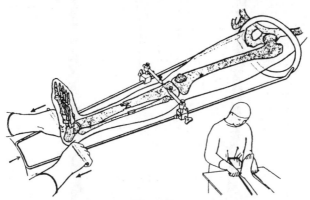

FIG. 183

Reduction of the fracture by traction. It must be emphasised
that once reduction is secured traction is removed; the nails are
left in position only to enhance fixation *not* to maintain traction.

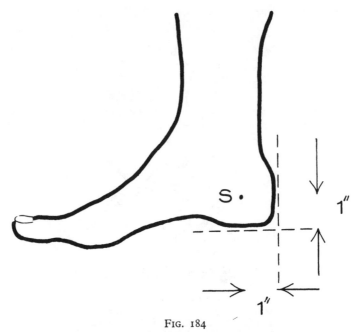

FIG. 184

Landmarks for avoiding transfixion of the subtaloid joint when inserting
a nail through the os calcis. Measurements are estimated from the
profile of the skin of the heel, as seen in side view.

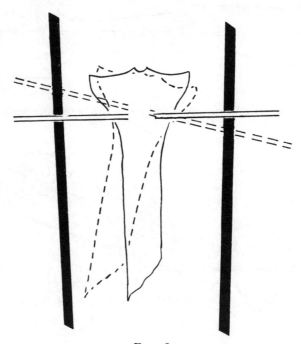

FIG. 185

Controlling varus and valgus alignment of the proximal
tibial fragment in McKee's method by altering the level
of attachment of the clamps on the side bars of the splint.

nail. The best landmark is a point 1 inch above and in front of the profile of the heel (Fig. 184). In order to avoid an erroneous position of rotation of the foot when this nail is clamped to the side bars of the splint, it is important that the assistant should hold the foot vertical while the surgeon is inserting the Stein-mann nail and taking care to keep the nail horizontal.

(2) Control of the proximal fragment. In controlling the alignment of the fractured tibia the distal fragment aligns itself with the axis of the splint and cannot be directly controlled because it is mobile on the ankle joint. The proximal fragment must be aligned by controlling its direction in the following way : *Valgus and varus angulation* is controlled by altering the level of attachment of the outer ends of this nail to the side bars of the splint. Thus by moving the lateral clamp proximally and the medial clamp distally, the proximal fragment will be directed in a valgus direction and vice versa (Fig. 185).

Forward and backward angulation is controlled by raising or lowering the knee and lower third of the thigh in relation to the Thomas splint. By means of a flannel sling and pad under the lower third of the thigh the proximal tibial fragment can be directed backwards by elevating the knee and forwards by allowing the knee to sag.

An extreme example of the salvage of a ' de-gloved ' leg, associated with a trans-verse fracture of the tibia and fibula, is illustrated in Fig. 186. The patient was a youth of twenty who had been run over by a bus and the opposite leg had evidence of threatened circulatory damage due to crushing of the calf muscles. This rendered it more than ever imperative that some attempt should be made to save the de-gloved leg. Even a below-knee amputation would not have been an immediate solution of the problem because it would have left a stump requiring a skin graft.

Having removed crushed muscles, cleaned the flap and removed fat, the skin was loosely sutured back in position and the whole limb splinted in the McKee apparatus. It was nursed with the skin exposed to the air and the limb supported in slings from behind. The skin flap died *in toto*, but by permitting it to become dry by exposure to the air no spreading infection developed. After three weeks the whole skin flap was black and hard. There was sensation in the foot and a good circulation, and the fracture was in good position.

Under anæsthesia the dry, black, skin cover was stripped away to leave a clean granulating surface covering all the muscles (Fig. 187). Postage stamp skin grafts were then applied at intervals of one week and the leg was nursed by exposure to the air under a protective cradle (Fig. 188).

The final state of healing of the leg is indicated in Figs. 189 and 190. The foot became grossly deformed because the forefoot had been permitted to fall into equinus (the extensor muscles having been largely removed at the time of the debridement) but this was later corrected by a wedge tarsectomy. The knee recovered a range of motion of 70 degrees. The opposite leg developed a Volkmann contracture of the calf, for which operations were necessary to correct the equinus deformity.

It is difficult to think of any other method by which such a limb could have been treated.

239

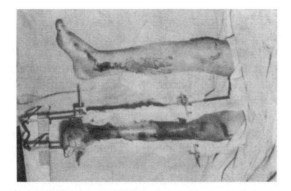

FIG. 186

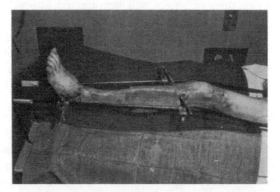

FIG. 187

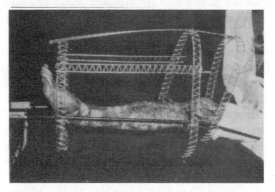

FIG. 188

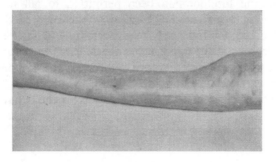

FIG. 189

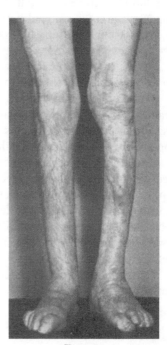

FIG. 190

Fig. 186—'De-gloved' left leg, with fracture of shaft of the tibia, treated by exposure to air in McKee's method.

Fig. 187—Same case about one month later when dead skin separated, leaving a granulating surface.

Fig. 188—First stage of skin-grafting by 'postage stamp' grafts. Note framework to permit leg to be nursed without dressings and with exposure to air continuously.

Fig. 189—State of healing of the grafts after six months.

Fig. 190—Result two years later.

Common Causes of Failure

While the McKee method of treating severe fractures of the tibia enables the position of the fragments to be controlled better than any other simple method, the technique still requires considerable skill and very careful observation. I have noticed from the work of my assistants that failure to get the best out of this method can usually be traced to one or other of the following facts :

1. Failure to control the position by failing to inspect the external contour of the limb.

2. Failure to inspect the contour of the limb as the result of covering the leg in plaster or bandages and failing to remove these for inspection during the first three weeks. It is possible to have an acceptable radiological picture with one tibial fragment pressing up through the skin ; what originally was a closed fracture may become compound with an ugly bony projection at the level of the fracture.

3. Failure to readjust the fragments, under anæsthesia, on one or two occasions during the first two weeks after the injury. There is a tendency to hope that the fragments will stay in perfect position without touching the apparatus after the primary treatment. The control of the fragments in this method is not complete, but the method has the advantage over other simple methods that it is possible to make minor adjustments without completely disturbing the fracture.

4. Failure to realise that the position of the proximal fragment is to some extent controlled by support under the lower end of the thigh.

Skeletal Traction : Os Calcis versus Tibia

In McKee's method traction applied through the os calcis is much better than traction through the lower end of the tibia. In passing a Steinmann nail through the lower end of the tibia the surgeon may have the misfortune of splitting the tibia if he chooses too high a level above the expanded lower end. If the nail is passed through the lower end of the tibia, on applying traction the bones will pull apart and yet continually return to their displaced position on removing the traction. This is caused by the tension of the posterior calf muscles and particularly those inserted into the tendo Achillis. If skeletal traction is applied to the lower end of the tibia the fragments will lift away from each other rather like the opening of the Tower Bridge (Fig. 191). The posterior muscles are not elongated by the traction force when it acts in the axis of the tibia. If the skeletal traction is applied to the os calcis the traction force acts directly in the axis of the calf muscles and, as these are the primary cause of the shortening, the fragments of the tibia will float into alignment.

Fracture of the Tibia associated with Fractures of the Femur

When both the tibia and the femur are fractured the problem is simplified by using internal fixation of one or other bone. If one of these bones is severely comminuted then the other will be chosen for internal fixation. The case illustrated in Fig. 192 had an extremely comminuted fracture of the lower third of the femur combined with a comminuted fracture of the tibia in which it was considered that internal fixation was unsuitable for both fractures. The McKee method of external skeletal fixation offered a useful solution to this problem.

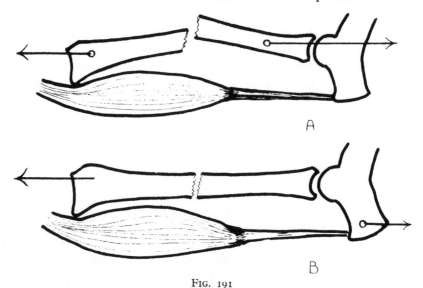

FIG. 191

Traction through the os calcis produces better alignment of tibial fractures than does traction to the lower end of the tibia.

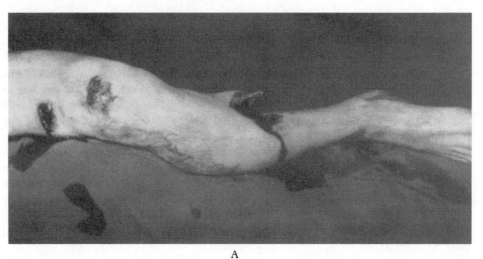

A

FIG. 192

Example of compound comminuted fractures of the lower third of the femur and midshaft of the tibia treated by McKee's method (see text).

Example.—The fracture of the femoral shaft was aligned first, by using the counter-traction of the ring of the splint against the root of the limb and applying temporary manual traction to the tibial nail. A pad and slings were placed behind the popliteal fossa and distal fragment of the femur. The tibial nail was then locked to the side bars of the Thomas splint using the McKee clamps. It was then possible to forget the femoral fracture and transfer all attention to the reduction of the tibial fracture. The final arrange-

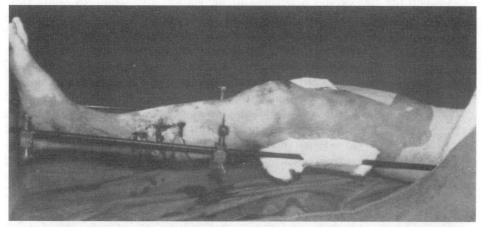

B

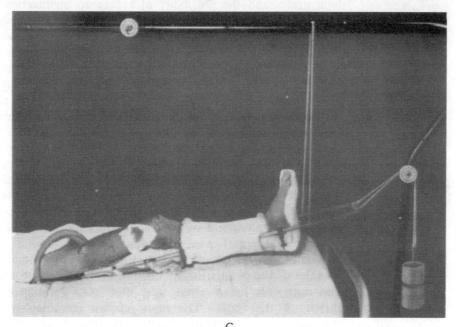

C

FIG. 192

Example of compound comminuted fractures of the lower third of the femur and midshaft of the tibia treated by McKee's method (see text).

ment of the splint is seen in Fig. 192, C, where a sliding traction force of 7 lb. was applied to the foot of the splint merely to make the arrangement more comfortable for the patient by reducing the pressure of the splint ring against the groin. A better arrangement would be to arrange a complete floating counterpoise for the whole splint.

THE BONE GRAFTING OF DELAYED UNION IN THE TIBIA

Though this monograph is devoted to the conservative treatment of fractures it is important to discuss the technique of bone grafting because the knowledge that there exists a certain safe and simple method of bone grafting has an important bearing on the planning of the initial treatment of recent fractures of the tibia. If a cortical bone graft, cut from the normal tibia and applied as an ' onlay ' to the un-united fracture by the Albee technique, were to be the only technique, no surgeon would contemplate such a major procedure unless a full period of conservative treatment in walking plaster, or caliper splint, had shown that spontaneous union was impossible. The same applies with equal force to the use of ' sliding ' tibial grafts which do not necessitate interference with the opposite tibia. If the original fracture has been compound and infected, prolonged delay—of at least six months—is essential when using massive tibial bone grafts, and the possibility of a flare-up of infection is still possible even several years after infected compound fractures. A recrudescence of infection when using a massive tibial onlay is a catastrophe of the first magnitude, because a cortical graft becomes an infected sequestrum with a very doubtful chance of being retained in the leg (Fig. 193) ; and to have violated the good tibia (with a 10 per cent. risk of spontaneous fracture in the donor leg) is a poor exchange for a sequestrating graft and the persistence of non-union.

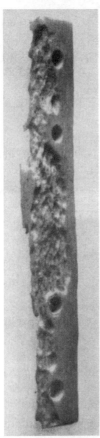

Fig. 193

Cortical bone-graft by Albee technique extracted one year after infected operation. Note erosion of the dead graft by granulation tissue. This graft acted as a sequestrum and healing of the wound did not take place until it was extracted.

Excluding the catastrophic result of infection in a graft of cortical bone, a little consideration shows that this type of graft cannot be justified biologically or mechanically. Biologically, cortical bone is not ' osteogenic ' because the sole source of osteogenesis is the living bone on which it is applied. It is a waste of valuable autogenous bone to have 75 per cent. of the graft situated remotely from the level of the pseudarthrosis instead of concentrating the grafted bone on all sides of the pseudarthrosis. Mechanically, a cortical bone graft can never be as strong as a steel plate forming one-quarter of the bulk. The most efficient combination of mechanical fixation with a bone graft, theoretically, would therefore be to use a plate for fixation, and chips of cancellous bone to surround the level of the pseudarthrosis to make an *artificial ensheathing callus.*

Naughton Dunn (1939) showed that in non-union of the tibia, when there was no loss of bone, and therefore no large gap between the ends of the bones, it was unnecessary to use a bone graft. By using a mallet and chisel he elevated the periosteum from the pseudarthrosis so that chips of cortex remained adherent to the periosteum. He called this technique his 'subcortical procedure,' and great care was taken not to strip the periosteum from the surface of the tibia before elevating these chips. The fracture line was occasionally curetted and the medullary canal opened up, but no graft was applied and the limb was merely immobilised in a plaster cast for three months. Jackson Burrows (1940), reporting on the technique taught by R. C. Elmslie, declared that it was unnecessary, and even harmful, to resect the bone ends or otherwise 'refresh' the fracture (which was popular at that time), and in this technique an inlaid cortical bone graft cut from the opposite tibia was applied across the line of the pseudarthrosis without otherwise disturbing it. It is, however, to D. B. Phemister (1947) that we owe the first clear statement of what I believe can now be accepted as axiomatic in bone grafting for non-union :

1. That a fibrous union should not be broken down nor should the bone ends be 'refreshed' or resected. To do so merely removes whatever mechanical stability is already present.
2. That the radiotranslucent tissues between the bone ends of a pseudarthrosis will ossify spontaneously when induced to do so by a bone graft laid on the surfaces.
3. That rigid immobilisation of the graft by screws, etc., is unnecessary if the graft is laid subperiosteally on the surface of the pseudarthrosis.
4. That such a subperiosteal graft can be used in the presence of recent sepsis if inserted through normal tissues away from the site of the original wound or sinus.

The technique of the Phemister bone graft can be improved by adding the 'subcortical' procedure of Naughton Dunn and by using slices of autogenous cancellous bone taken from the iliac crest in place of the cortical bone used by Phemister. Using this technique the procedure is so simple and efficacious that it can be used as early as three months after a fracture—i.e., in 'delayed union' rather than in true 'non-union.' It can be used in recently infected fractures because even if it becomes infected itself the major part of the cancellous bone will survive and no sequestrum will be left behind because the infected part will either be dissolved away or extruded (Fig. 194).

The decision to graft can be made three months after a fracture of the tibia purely on the amount of movement which can be detected clinically. Little or no attention need be paid to the radiological appearance in making this decision. If there is only a trace of fibrous 'give' after three months of conservative treatment, so little in fact that quite careful attention is needed for it to be demonstrated, then spontaneous union in a further walking plaster or caliper splint can confidently be expected. If after three months of conservative treatment a fracture of the tibia shows a clearly detectable range of free motion, then an immediate Phemister graft is to be advised rather than perseverance with further plaster fixation.

The failure rate of the Phemister type of graft, if autogenous slices of iliac bone are used, is extremely small. One reason for this is that in accordance with the policy here advocated it is used 'prophylactically' and before the more difficult situation of true non-union has supervened. In a personal series of thirty cases there have been only three cases in which the graft was not completely solid when the plaster was removed three months after operation. One of these united later spontaneously, another was successfully treated by a second Phemister graft. The isolated failure was a case in which a large whole diameter segment of the tibia was completely ischæmic at the time of grafting (Fig. 159, p. 207).

I am indebted to D. B. Forbes [1] for analysing the results of my series of Phemister bone grafts as applied to the tibia. The infected cases are of particular interest. Thirty patients submitted to grafting included five who had a discharging sinus at the time of the operation and four in whom the wound developed infection

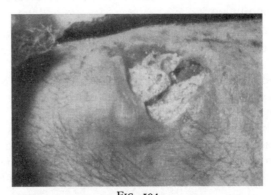

FIG. 194

Gross example of the infection of an autogenous iliac bone-graft when inserted into an infected compound fracture. Three dead fragments extruded spontaneously but the underlying fragments, four or five in number, were successfully incorporated and the fracture united. This procedure would be totally unjustifiable if an autogenous cortical bone-graft had been used.

though the compound tibial fracture appeared to have been sterile at the time of the operation. All nine of these infected cases united though one required a second graft by reason of the fact that 1 inch of bone had been lost from the tibial diaphysis at the original injury. In three patients the original sinus was healed by the time the plaster was removed after the graft. In six patients the fracture was united and the patients bearing weight before final healing of the wound occurred. In these severely compound cases the average interval between injury and union was fourteen months but in the cases where grafting was performed within twenty weeks of the injury the average time between injury and union was eight months.

These figures are the results over a period of twelve years during which I was gaining experience in this method and before the full value of the technique was realised. Very few of these cases were grafted under six months. By adopting the policy of grafting earlier, *i.e.*, about three months after the fracture, I feel certain

[1] In press.

that these figures could be greatly improved and that no serious hazard would be incurred as a result of early grafting.

Technique

Certain details of the technique need to be emphasised. The operation is essentially a *subcortical* procedure, the periosteum being raised with a hammer and chisel so as to produce ' shingles ' of cortical bone adherent to it. The idea is to construct an *artificial ensheathing callus*.

A straight longitudinal incision is made in the line of the subcutaneous border of the tibia and centred over the fracture line. The incision is deepened directly to bone throughout the length of the wound, *avoiding any undercutting of the subcutaneous tissues* which are usually indurated and adherent to the subjacent periosteum.

A sharp chisel is now used and, taking care not to strip the periosteum from the underlying bone, thin chips or shingles of cortical bone are elevated so that the periosteum is turned up as an osteoperiosteal flap. This procedure is adopted on the subcutaneous and the lateral surfaces of the tibia but no attempt is made to reach the posterior surface (Fig. 195, A). At the end of this stage it will be seen that two deep gutters have been produced, both lined with adherent bone chips. It will be immediately obvious that if these gutters were to be packed with slices of iliac bone they would be held open and it would be impossible to approximate the edges of the wound. This difficulty in closure is rendered the more so because the surrounding soft tissues are indurated and inelastic. To facilitate closure it is important to pass the chisel through the floor of the groove, using it as a lever against the fulcrum of the tibia to split open the deepest part of the groove (Fig. 195, B). This will mean tearing the periosteum and fibrous tissue in the region of the postero-medial and postero-lateral angles of the tibia. With tissue forceps attached to the edges of the wound, traction is applied to the osteoperiosteal walls of the gutter, and by palpating with the finger any tight fibrous structures can be discovered which are preventing them from being mobilised. Time spent in mobilising the osteoperiosteal structures sufficiently to allow easy closure after the iliac bone has been inserted will be well worth while.

Iliac bone slices, 2 to 3 mm. thick, are now cut from the iliac crest and laid on the surfaces of the tibia and the wound drawn together (Fig. 195, C). Closure is in one layer, using skin sutures alone. I think it is important to insist that the iliac bone should be in the form of flexible strips at least 2½ inches long. Small chips of bone are not reliable by themselves because a pseudarthrosis line can form between them. It is impossible to close the osteoperiosteal flaps separately (nor is it desirable). The use of an interrupted vertical stitch is recommended for this closure in one layer (Fig. 195, D).

Plaster is then applied over the wool, care being taken to split the plaster longitudinally. In the subsequent twenty-four hours there is invariably a considerable expansion of this split, showing that its omission might have caused pain and perhaps dangerous circulatory embarrassment (Fig. 196).

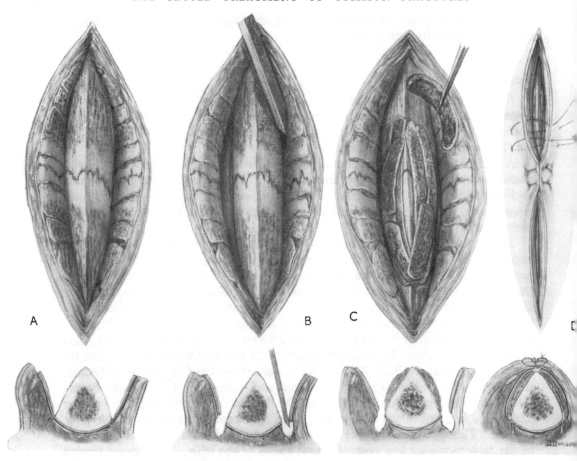

FIG. 195
Stages in the Phemister bone graft
A, Subcortical exposure in one layer.
B, Opening the posterior gutter to mobilise the osteoperiosteal flaps.
C, Applying the iliac bone slices.
D, Closure in one layer, skin alone.

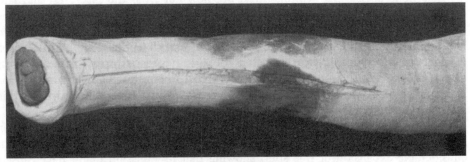

FIG. 196
Plaster split immediately after application. Note gaping of the split within first twelve hours.

This plaster is left untouched for six weeks, during which time the patient can be ambulatory but non-weight-bearing on crutches. The plaster is then changed, the stitches removed, and a close-fitting walking plaster applied for a further six weeks. Usually the tibia will be found clinically solid six weeks after operation when the first plaster is changed, and three months after operation it will be possible to allow the start of full function without plaster and *before radiological consolidation of the shaft of the tibia is proved* (Fig. 197). By permitting weight-bearing when clinical union is present, irrespective of radiological appearances, no case in my series of thirty patients later developed movement or pseudarthrosis.

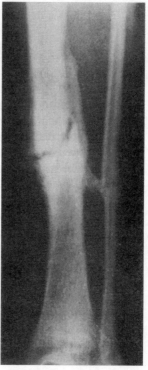

Special Note

I must emphasise that *strips* of cancellous bone are superior to chips or small fragments of cancellous bone in this method of grafting. When small chips of bone are used it is possible for these to fuse into two or three conglomerations with a fibrous union forming between the main masses. This possibility of failure does not occur when relatively long slices of iliac bone are laid on the surface of the bone.

Fig. 197—Typical result of Phemister graft three months after operation. Clinically solid though radiologically tibial fracture still visible. Patient permitted full weight-bearing without plaster.

FIG. 197

REFERENCES

BURROWS, H. JACKSON (1940). *Proc. R. Soc. Med.*, **33**, 157.
COMPERE, E. L. (1949). *J. Bone Jt Surg.*, **31**, 47.
DUNN, NAUGHTON (1939). Treatment of un-united fracture. *Brit. med. J.*, **2**, 221.
GROVES, E. W. HEY (1921). *Modern Methods of Treating Fractures.* Bristol : Wright.
PHEMISTER, D. B. (1947). *J. Bone Jt Surg.*, **29**, 946.
URIST, M. R., MAZET, ROBERT, Jun. & McLEAN, F. C. (1954). *J. Bone Jt Surg.*, **36A**, 931.

CHAPTER SIXTEEN

THE POTT'S FRACTURE

THE precision with which it is possible to reduce a Pott's fracture by manipulation becomes a source of pleasure once the surgeon understands the mechanics of this reduction. My own satisfaction is increased when I recall the uncertainty of my own early attempts to reduce this fracture-dislocation and how I was once dependent on the X-ray as on a ' lucky dip.'

The problem in treating a Pott's fracture is not so much how to reduce the fracture but how to make sure that it will stay reduced. I shall endeavour to indicate when I think it is dangerous to persist with closed reduction and when operative aid should be invoked.

Operative treatment of the Pott's fracture is not a procedure to be encouraged as a routine, because there are special complications of operative treatment quite as serious as the defects of closed treatment. In the ordinary Pott's fracture the functional and anatomical results of a skilful closed reduction should be perfect. Even if a small posterior marginal fragment remains displaced, the ankle possesses a latitude for recovery of function which is often astonishing. The open reduction of this fracture-dislocation can be a matter of considerable technical difficulty; to secure adequate exposure in the cramped space available may impair the blood supply of a detached fragment. If for any reason open reduction should be attempted, nothing less than a ' hair-line ' restoration should be regarded as justifying it; incomplete reduction after open operation must be regarded as an error of judgment. If open reduction is considered imperative, then the minimum of metallic ' hardware ' should be used. An injured ankle is prone to chronic œdema, and as it has no muscle covering it is subject to extreme temperature changes, which I believe can cause pain when screw-heads are lying close to the subcutaneous tissues.

THE ANATOMY OF THE POTT'S FRACTURE

There have been various attempts to classify ankle fractures according to the different types of violence producing the fracture but these classifications do not offer help in treatment.

The common fracture-dislocation of the ankle joint, called the Pott's fracture or sometimes the ' third-degree abduction-external-rotation fracture,' is composed of three separate fractures combined with a postero-lateral dislocation of the ankle joint. The three fractures involve the medial and lateral malleoli and the so-called ' third malleolus,' which is a posterior marginal fragment of the articular surface of the tibia. In a severely displaced fracture the X-ray may present an appearance of utter confusion, and the student may well feel that he will be very lucky indeed to get even one of these ' malleoli ' reduced, let alone three at the same time ! This erroneous conception springs from concentrating on the radiological appearances of the individual fragments without understanding the anatomy of the injury as a whole (Fig. 38, p. 44).

In reality this complicated fracture consists only of two parts (Fig. 198) : a proximal part, represented by the shafts of the tibia and the fibula, and a distal part, represented by the whole *foot*. The crux of this reduction is the knowledge that **the astragalus, the medial malleolus, the third malleolus, and the lateral malleolus all move as one piece,** being inseparably connected by the ligaments of the ankle joint. *Reduction of the displacement is therefore secured by concentrating on the displacement of the astragalus in relation to the tibia rather than making any*

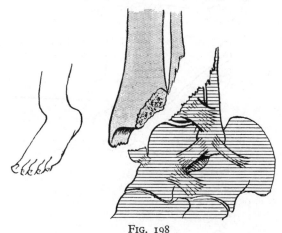

Fig. 198

Anatomy of the Pott's fracture. Showing how the foot together with all the distal fragments move as one unit while the proximal fragments consist only of the shafts of the tibia and fibula.

local attack on one or other of the malleoli. In practice, therefore, the act of reduction merely consists of restoring the alignment of the foot to the axis of the leg. In doing this the sense of touch, by which the sensation of reduction is most often obtained, can be enhanced by a good eye for subtle distortions of outline ; indeed a shrewd observer can often guess from the external shape of a plaster whether a reduction has been obtained or not. One of my own visual landmarks in this reduction concerns the projection of the heel behind the line of the sub-cutaneous border of the tibia ; the horizontal distance between these is increased with posterior displacement of the foot.

The Use of Gravity in Reduction

The importance of recognising the role of gravity in producing deformity is nowhere better illustrated than in the special example of the Pott's fracture. It cannot be too often emphasised that **to assess the effect of gravity on a**

251

displacement while the patient is under anæsthesia is as much part of any reduction as is a knowledge of the effects of muscular tone when the patient is conscious.

If the leg is held in the horizontal position supported only under the calf and

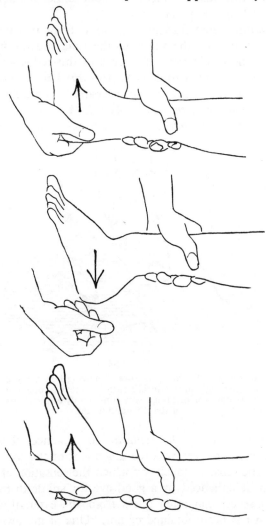

FIG. 199

Exploring the range of anteroposterior displacement
before applying the plaster. Assessing the influence of
gravity in causing redisplacement.

without any support below the foot, a Pott's fracture will fall into full posterior displacement. In this position an important step in the reduction consists of *assessing the range of the excursion from the position of maximum posterior displacement to the position of reduction* (Fig. 199). By committing this range to memory the surgeon obtains a mental picture which will help him in a later stage of the reduction. In a similar way *the range of mobility between the position of maximal lateral displacement and full reduction should also be assessed* and remembered (Fig. 200).

By exploring the mobility of the Pott's fracture in this way it will soon become evident that a reduction can be obtained, and can be held, without using force and merely by using gravity and the weight of the foot. **By holding the foot in one hand with the heel resting in the palm, with the foot and leg held horizontally and in external rotation, the ankle will fall spontaneously into**

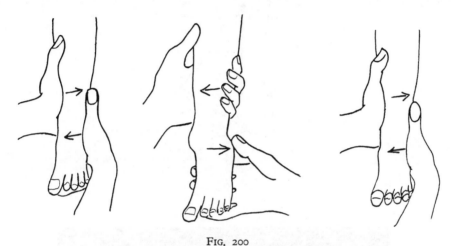

FIG. 200

Exploring the range of lateral displacement between the maximum deformity and the position of apparent reduction.

the position of reduction (Fig. 201, A, B). It is only when the surgeon understands how unnecessary is the use of muscular violence that he really appreciates the mechanics of the Pott's fracture.

From the emphasis laid on the synergic use of gravity in this reduction it is hardly necessary to draw attention to the fact that the preceding mechanism, *i.e.*, supporting the foot behind the heel, must never be used in those rarer types of ankle fracture with *anterior* displacement of the talus. In these cases the reverse position must be used and the foot must be allowed to fall backwards under its own weight by supporting the leg behind the calf alone. This illustrates how important it is not to reduce any fracture by ritual movements but to assess the influence of various mechanical factors on each injury as an individual case.

The Elimination of Gravity

Some surgeons instead of using gravity to give positive help in the reduction just described prefer to rearrange forces so that gravity is eliminated; in the Pott's fracture this can be done by carrying out the reduction with the tibia in the vertical position by hanging it over the end of a table. This is a good procedure and the surgeon can adopt it as a matter of personal inclination; the correction

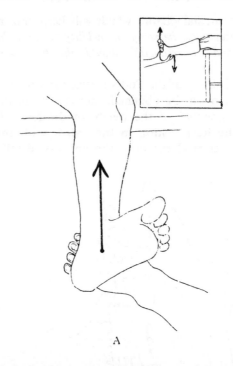

A

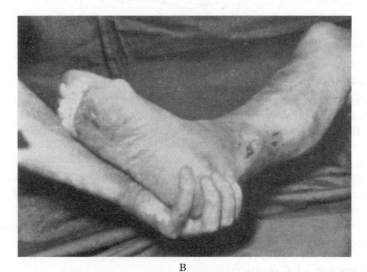

B

FIG. 201

Showing how gravity can be invoked to maintain reduction if the heel is supported while the *whole leg* and foot are allowed to fall into some degree of external rotation. This corrects the postero-lateral displacement of the foot on the leg. An assistant supports the knee.

254

of the postero-lateral displacement is carried out as just described, but in this position the surgeon's hands must exert pressure in the appropriate direction. The following technical details are applicable though the vertical method is not the one recommended here.

THE APPLICATION OF PLASTER

The Pott's fracture is best treated by the surgeon applying his own plaster; the surgeon alone appreciates the urgency of the situation and the absolute necessity for completing the plaster while it is still soft and before it has reached the consistency of damp cardboard to obscure his sense of touch.

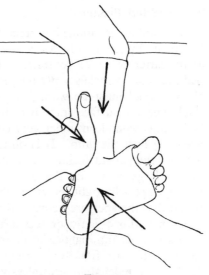

For the initial purpose of the reduction only sufficient plaster should be applied to be strong enough to hold the reduction temporarily when it has set; this is usually about three 8-inch bandages. During this application no attention should be paid to the ultimate finish of the upper and lower limits of the plaster, which would waste time and invite setting of the cast before the reduction has been obtained. During the rapid application of these three bandages it is unnecessary to keep the fracture either precisely reduced or the foot precisely at a right angle; it is enough for the assistant merely to *hold the foot by the toes*.

Having completed the speedy application of these three bandages the surgeon now takes the fracture from the assistant and 'feels' the fracture by moving it about inside the wet plaster; from his previous analysis of the fracture he should be able

FIG. 202

Position for moulding the plaster while setting. Note hands at different levels and *whole limb* in 45 degrees of external rotation (*i.e.,* knee externally rotated as well as foot).

again to recognise the sensation of reduction, though his tactile impressions will now be a little muffled by the plaster. Having recognised the sensation of reduction he now holds the reduction without further movement until the plaster has set; during this time he invokes the assistance of gravity with an assistant maintaining the foot and leg in external rotation while the surgeon supports the foot with his hand below the heel (Fig. 202). The plaster is now completed by finishing the top and bottom of the cast and applying extra bandages to increase the thickness if deemed necessary.

It will be seen from the foregoing that from the moment of completing the plaster no more than two or three movements are required to recapture the reduction; these **simple rehearsed movements** are **succeeded by a period of complete immobility.** Contrast this with what is seen when the beginner attempts his first reduction with inadequate instruction. After much struggling and muscular violence it is suspected that a reduction has probably been secured and the application of the plaster is then commenced. An assistant applies the plaster but is impeded in doing this by further last-minute attempts by the surgeon to 'improve' his reduction as new inspirations strike him. Impeded in his attempts to complete the plaster, the assistant applies a rough and irregular cast which is just hardening when the surgeon decides on a final change of tactics. Finally, all further attempts at improving the position being obviously futile, it is decided to see what sort of a position has been obtained by using the X-ray as a ' lucky dip.'

The Padded Plaster

If padding is applied correctly, it can actually *enhance* the fixation of the fragments by its slightly resilient action, which can adapt the plaster to the limb as the latter swells or contracts. This is quite contrary to the popular idea that padding always makes a plaster loose. To apply the padding correctly (Chapter V), the wool must be wound on, with very great care, in a layer about ½ inch thick, and the surface smoothed down before the plaster is applied. The plaster bandage is wound on under very considerable tension so as to compress the wool evenly against the limb. It is quite astonishing how much tension can be applied without the patient feeling any distress, because the pressure is evenly distributed over a large area. At the upper end of the plaster it is essential to pull the bandage specially tight, because otherwise, at the completion of the cast, it will be found that the aperture between the upper end of plaster and the calf is extremely capacious. For this reason it is *advisable to omit the wool in the proximal part.*

As regards the manner of finishing the plaster at the toes it is probably best to leave the toes free by stopping the plaster at the metatarso-phalangeal joints. A platform under the toes, unless very carefully made, often produces a cocked-up position.

THREE COMMON SOURCES OF ERROR IN REDUCING THE POTT'S FRACTURE

There are three points in reducing this fracture which are often not adequately appreciated ; they are of great importance in making it possible for the surgeon practically to guarantee a complete manipulative reduction of a fresh fracture.

1. Keeping the Foot at Right Angles to the Leg

In the commendable desire to maintain the fully plantigrade position of the foot during the hardening of the plaster, forceful dorsiflexion is often produced by pressure applied to the sole of the forefoot. This method of causing dorsiflexion can cause a relapse of the posterior displacement of the talus. When difficulty is experienced in getting the foot to the right angle (as when the tendo Achillis is short) by upward pressure against the sole of the forefoot, the pivotal point will move away from the ankle joint and pass to the insertion of the tendo Achillis (Fig. 203, A) (in other words, from being a lever of the first degree it becomes a lever of the second degree). With the pivot at the insertion of the tendo Achillis into the heel, **dorsiflexion, by force applied to the sole of the forefoot, will push the talus out of the ankle mortice posteriorly.**

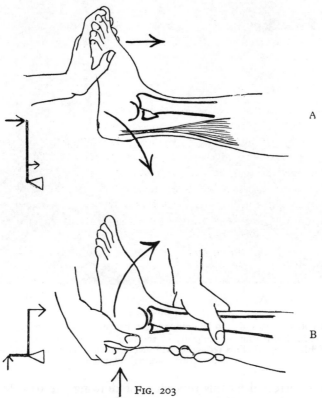

FIG. 203

A, Showing the disastrous effect of struggling to secure a plantigrade foot, especially if the tendo Achillis is tight, by forcing the forefoot upwards. This pushes the talus out of the ankle joint posteriorly by the system of levers illustrated.

B, Showing how the plantigrade position should be obtained by lifting the heel forwards—dorsiflexing the forefoot through the medium of the system of levers illustrated. This method enhances the security of the reduction.

It is possible to produce dorsiflexion of the foot without invoking posterior displacement, by exerting the dorsiflexion force indirectly through the heel instead of directly through the forefoot. **To dorsiflex the foot correctly, the hand which supports the heel should draw the os calcis downwards and forwards so as to bring the hindfoot into the plantigrade position** (Fig. 203, B). This movement greatly assists the reduction by pulling the talus forwards. If, now, the forefoot is still in some degree of plantar flexion, owing to dropping at the mid-tarsal joint, it is permissible to apply some gentle upward pressure to the sole of the forefoot by resting it against the surgeon's chest; this will have no ill effect provided that control of the heel is maintained by the hand which grips it. The example illustrated in Fig. 204 shows how a defective initial

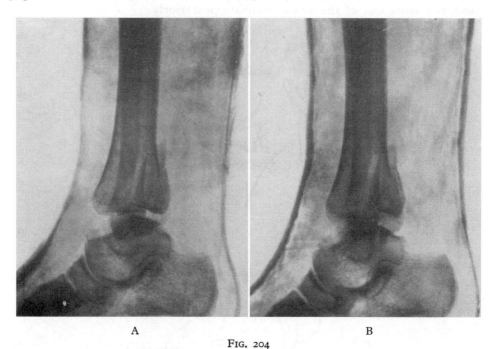

A   B

FIG. 204

A, Unreduced Pott's fracture due to ignorance of mechanism explained in Fig. 203, A.
B, Successful reduction (as far as congruity of the talus with axis of tibia is concerned) by using the method of Fig. 203, B. This reduction will give a satisfactory result even with this unreduced posterior marginal fragment.

reduction was corrected by this procedure of drawing the os calcis forwards and downwards.

2. Compressing the Mortice

This phrase is often used to denote an attempt to reduce diastasis of the tibio-fibular joint by compressing the malleoli towards each other and narrowing the width of the ankle joint. This attempt is prone to failure if the obvious attack by direct compression of the two malleoli is adopted. The reason for this is that the force of compression applied to the malleoli is wasted on the soft tissues in a swollen ankle. If the ankle is swollen, **simple side-to-side compression merely applies the same pressure to each side of the talus, which therefore remains in the displaced position having no urge to move more to one side than the other** (Fig. 205, A).

To secure medial movement of the displaced talus, and with it medial movement of the external malleolus, the forces applied to the ankle must be applied

258

at different levels. **The pressure applied to the outer side of the foot must be below the external malleolus and the pressure applied to the inner side of the ankle must be above the medial malleolus.** Under these conditions the talus will have high pressure on the outer side and low pressure

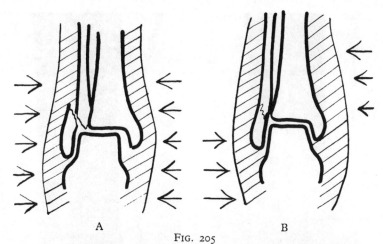

A   B

FIG. 205

A, Showing how the attempt to 'narrow the mortice' by applying a 'squeezing' grip with the hands at the same level over each malleolus fails to move the talus because equal pressure is exerted both sides of it.

B, Showing how the talus moves into position, taking the external malleolus with it, when pressures are exerted at different levels.

on the inner side and will therefore move towards the medial malleolus *even in the presence of gross swelling* of the ankle (Fig. 205, B).

In Fig. 206, A and B, is seen a failure to reduce the widening of an ankle when a faulty technique was used and also the reduction obtained when the correct method was used. Note here the moulding of the plaster at the levels of maximum pressure situated above and below the plane of movement of the fracture.

3. Rotation

Failure to observe the correct rotatory alignment of the foot to the tibia, as shown by the alignment of the toes and patella, is a common source of incomplete reduction. The Pott's fracture has an external rotation element in the force which originally produced the deformity, and it is therefore essential to *keep the foot internally rotated during the reduction and application of the plaster.* External rotation of the talus carries the external malleolus posteriorly and tends to perpetuate the displacement of the external malleolus which is so commonly seen in the lateral film (Fig. 207, A). Probably some interposition of soft parts occurs in this displacement of the external malleolus because it commonly resists attempts at perfect reduction; however, slight displacement as seen in the lateral view seems to cause no disability if the talus is well reduced in relation to the articular surface of the tibia.

The importance of rotation in widening the mortice becomes obvious when one recollects that the talus is square in its horizontal section ; any rotation from its normal position will therefore tend to widen the mortice by forcing the malleoli apart (Fig. 207, B). Therefore in holding the *leg* in external rotation,

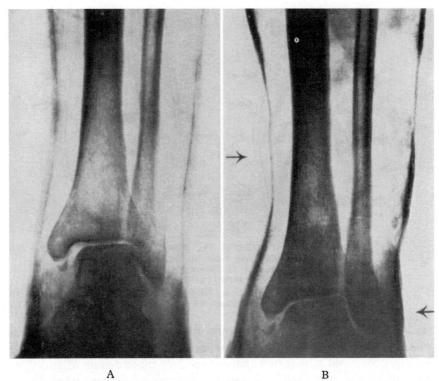

A   B

FIG. 206

A, Faulty reduction when the mortice was compressed from side to side by pressure at equal levels.

B, Mortice now congruous. Note the shape of the plaster marking the site of the pressure applied above and below the fracture level.

as instructed on page 254 (Fig. 201), it is important to *see that the foot is in very slight internal rotation.*

Fear of Over-reduction

Incomplete reduction of a Pott's fracture can often be traced to a subconscious fear on the part of the operator that he might displace the talus and the associated medial malleolus too far medially. A good example of this is seen in Fig. 208 where the operator at the first reduction deliberately refrained from applying maximal pressure and did in fact try the manœuvre of ' compressing the mortice,' which has been criticised in Fig. 206. At the second reduction, where the operator's force was directed in a three-point system, the reduction is seen to

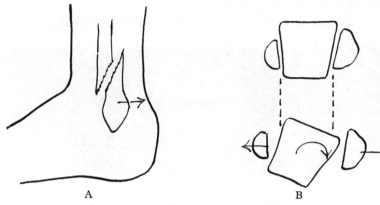

FIG. 207

A, Posterior displacement of the external malleolus probably due to external rotation.

B, Showing the effect of rotation of the talus in separating the malleoli. Knee and foot must therefore always be in correct rotary relation during reduction.

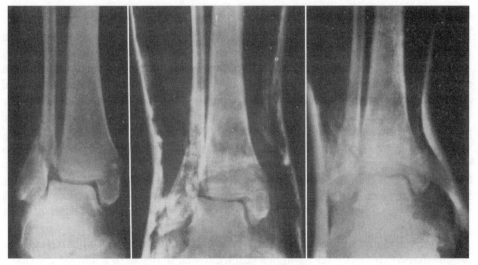

FIG. 208

Example of faulty reduction due to fear of over-correction. The operator 'compressed the mortice' with hands at same level (Fig. 205). Note good reduction by forcing correction to maximum. Note modelling of plaster above and below level of ankle joint.

261

be complete. Note the different modelling of the plaster in the last, successful, reduction compared with the preceding plaster.

One of the very few cases of true over-reduction which I have ever seen is

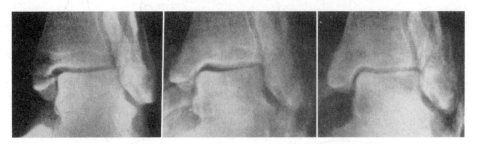

FIG. 209

A rare case of over-correction. Patient instructed to bear weight during first week and perfect reduction obtained spontaneously.

illustrated in Fig. 209, but it is also interesting to observe that a spontaneous correction was obtained simply by allowing the patient to bear weight during the first week.

X-RAY CRITERIA IN THE ANKLE JOINT

1. The Anteroposterior View

Gross degrees of widening of the ankle mortice are readily recognised, but the student will often have difficulty in satisfying himself in minor degrees of displacement. In the normal ankle it is impossible to see a clear gap between the talus and both malleoli in any one film (except a tomogram). In the standard anteroposterior position a clear view is visible through the space between the talus and the medial malleolus, but a varying degree of overlap in the external malleolus is always present. The essential feature is to recognise the normal width of the gap between the talus and the medial malleolus. This gap varies slightly in different normal subjects—in most cases it is equal to the gap between the lower surface of the tibia and the upper surface of the talus, but in others the space between the tibia above and the talus below is a shade narrower than the medial gap, probably due to atrophy of weight-bearing cartilage in older persons.

In the anteroposterior radiograph it is useful to note that the talus has a slight saddle-shaped concavity on its upper surface which mates with a similar convexity on the lower end of the tibia. If these saddle-shaped surfaces are in register one can presume that the main articulation is reduced regardless of the position of the medial malleolus.

A point which frequently gives rise to suspicion and worry is an appearance of tibio-fibular diastasis. If the amount is so slight that it is doubtful, then it is not important **provided that the talus and the medial malleolus are in**

262

normal contact. The appearance of widening of the tibio-fibular synostosis may be due to swelling and œdema of the damaged tibio-fibular ligament, and all attempts to reduce such small degrees of diastasis will fail if the medial malleolus is already in its normal site. In these cases I feel certain that the malleolus usually settles in place again as the swollen ligament contracts and heals.

2. The Lateral View

It has been stated in a previous paragraph that, with reasonable dexterity and knowledge, the surgeon should almost be able to guarantee a perfect reduction by close methods in most fresh ankle fractures. This is true with two exceptions: (1) gross separation of the medial malleolus, and (2) upward displacement of a posterior marginal fragment. Both these complications may suggest the necessity for open operation.

As regards upward displacement of a 'posterior marginal fragment,' it is the exception rather than the rule to influence its position by closed reduction, and it therefore remains to decide how important, if at all, is some permanent residual displacement of this fragment.

The essential feature about a posterior marginal fracture is not the amount of displacement but the *size* of the displaced fragment; and the essential feature about the size of the displaced fragment is its effect in inviting redisplacement of the talus if it comprises more than one-third of the anteroposterior diameter of the articular surface. **If the talus can be retained in complete congruity with the anterior part of the articular surface of the tibia the ankle joint will in all probability give an excellent functional result** even if the posterior marginal fragment is widely displaced. This is not as surprising as might at first appear when it is remembered that the lateral radiograph of the ankle does not generally represent the true state of the lower surface of the tibia. The posterior marginal fragment is never separated by a transverse fracture line; the fracture line is always oblique and the 'marginal' fragment is merely the separation of a postero-lateral *corner* from the articular

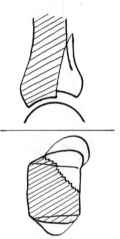

FIG. 210

Showing that the appearance seen in the lateral view (*see also* Fig. 204, B) is not incompatible with a good functional result because the fracture is not transverse and the defect of the articular surface only concerns one corner. Provided that the talus is congruous with the shaft of the tibia (*see* Fig. 211, B) a good result is likely even if the posterior marginal fragment is considerably displaced.

surface (Fig. 210). There is usually, therefore, enough articular surface of the tibia at the postero-medial surface to render the talus stable, and the actual state is not as bad as the X-ray might at first suggest. An apparent 'step' on the articular surface of the tibia will not present a ridge to the talus because the step will fill with fibrocartilage and the talus will still operate against a smooth surface. If, however, the talus is allowed to slip backwards by even a fraction of an inch a more serious state of affairs will exist than would result from the mere loss of articular area as represented by the displaced posterior fragment. *If the surface of the talus is not congruous with the anterior surface of the intact part of the tibia it will bear against the posterior edge of this articular surface and so produce a pressure* ' high spot ' subject to the whole of the body weight, and osteo-arthritis will commence.

This example illustrates an important mechanical principle ; **complete congruity of the unfractured part of a joint is better than improving the**

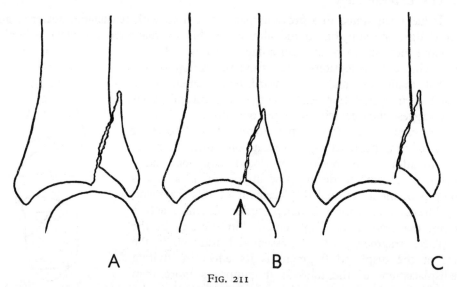

FIG. 211

Illustrating how it is better to leave posterior fragment fully displaced, *provided that* the main tibio-talar articulation is congruous (C), rather than ' improve ' the position of the displaced fragment and leave the main articulation slightly subluxed (B). Note ' high spot ' between talus and tibia in B.

position of the displaced fragment but leaving the main part of the joint slightly subluxed (Fig. 211).

THE THREE-POINT PLASTER

The reduction and fixation of the Pott's fracture is an excellent example of the three-point action of a plaster cast, the essential points of which are illustrated in Fig. 49, page 52.

Post-reduction Regime

In a fracture where there has been displacement of the talus no useful purpose is ever served by insisting on early weight-bearing. It is true that the articular platform of the tibia is horizontal, and theoretically there should be no force acting in a sideways direction to induce the talus to redisplace. But the ankle takes the whole weight of the body, and if weight-bearing is not allowed in fractures through the hip or the knee for eight weeks there is no reason why the ankle should be an exception. A severe Pott's fracture requires three months fixation in plaster of Paris. The first two months can be non-weight-bearing and the last month fully weight-bearing. In less severe fractures the period of non-weight-bearing can be reduced to one month. Fractures without displacement can bear weight from the start.

The total duration of plaster fixation can be assessed by that important detail mentioned previously in regard to the rehabilitation of any fracture in an ambulant plaster: it is pointless to remove a plaster at a fixed time if the patient is not walking energetically in that plaster and without a stick. If the patient is not walking briskly before the end of three months he is not receiving adequate rehabilitation and encouragement (and hence there is a psychic hold-up), or there is some complication, such as an extreme bone atrophy, or the plaster is a bad one and is uncomfortable. If the plaster is taken off before the patient is walking well he will walk even worse or possibly not at all.

Skeletal Traction in Pott's Fractures

Some surgeons frequently resort to skeletal traction in complicated Pott's fractures by applying traction through the os calcis with the limb on a Braun's splint.

When skill has been acquired in the manipulative reduction and plaster fixation of the Pott's fracture the number of cases needing skeletal traction will be very small; in my own experience I have rarely found the results of skeletal traction so much superior to manipulative measures to justify the longer hospital-isation needed by this method.

There is considerable danger of distracting the talus from contact with the tibia even with light traction in cases where there has been ligamentary damage.

CRITICISM OF OPERATIVE TREATMENT

There is a growing tendency to recommend open reduction and internal fixation of displaced fractures of the medial malleolus on the grounds that to hold the medial malleolus is the ' key ' to holding the whole reduction. Though there is much to be said in favour of this doctrine it is quite unnecessary to apply it as a routine, because so many Pott's fractures can be treated perfectly by closed methods throughout. I myself dislike the idea of the head of a screw lying in the fibres of the medial collateral ligament almost exactly at the centre of motion in this ligament. It is no difficult matter to remove a screw in this site when the fracture is united, but very few surgeons do this.

The common example of a diastasis of the ankle joint associated with a fracture of the external malleolus (Fig. 212) illustrates the importance of mastering the technique of closed reduction in preference to operative treatment. To insert a screw into a fracture of the external malleolus at a level as low as in this case would be difficult without endangering the articular surfaces of the joint. By modelling the plaster above and below the level of the ankle joint the diastasis can be held reduced.

I have not myself found any need to try internal fixation of the external malleolus by wire 'encirclage' and have mentioned the adverse biological effect of encirclage when applied to fractures in cortical bone (p. 26).

One of the peculiar dangers inherent in the operative treatment of ankle fractures is that a fragment can too easily be fixed in a position *where it ought not to be* and where it is positively harmful. The safety of the conservative method is that, provided the main articular surfaces of the talus and tibia are congruous, displaced fragments imperfectly reduced tend to lie out of the way and will not impinge

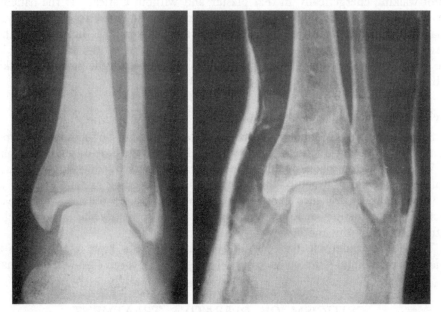

FIG. 212

Diastasis of ankle with low fracture of the external malleolus. Skilful plaster technique ought to hold this. To screw this low fracture might damage the ankle joint.

on the main articulations with harmful pressure. Thus in Fig. 213 the medial malleolus has been fixed too far in and will eventually be much more harmful than if it had been allowed to remain, un-united, a slight distance away from the talus. In Fig. 214 the operator was highly delighted with the result of screwing this tibio-fibular diastasis but did not notice that he had closed the mortice too much and that the talus was held away from the tibial surface. The end result, even after removing the screw, was the development of traumatic arthritis within two years. It is very difficult to decide how much to close the mortice of the ankle joint; if it is not closed sufficiently the operation was unnecessary; if it is closed too much it is harmful. *The talus fits the ankle mortice only in full dorsiflexion, so that in a large part of its ordinary range of movement, as when jumping on the toes, it is working in a mortice which is anatomically loose on the talus.*

When the displaced fragment of the medial malleolus is small it is unwise to use a screw. Fractures involving only the tip of the medial malleolus can be left displaced even if they become un-united. Not only may the screw produce comminution of the tip of the malleolus and produce non-union, but it is essential for the screw to be very vertical if it is to avoid entering the joint. This is often

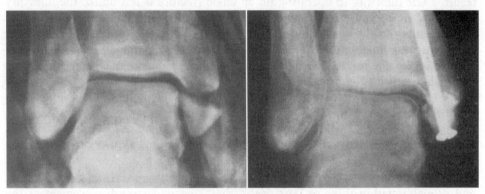

FIG. 213

Fracture of tip of medial malleolus. Position after operation is worse than a fibrous union in original position. Note that the head of the vertical screw lies entirely inside axis of movement of deltoid ligament. Screws placed less vertically, in larger fragments, lie away from the important axis of rotation in the ligament. A catgut stitch would have been better.

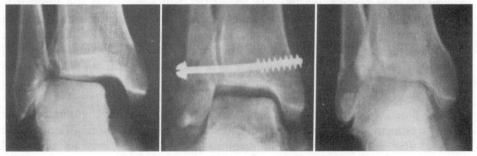

FIG. 214

Too enthusiastic closure of mortice in a diastasis. The talus cannot reach the articular surface of the tibia. Rapid onset of traumatic arthritis even after removal of screw.

technically difficult, and in any case this vertical position puts the screw-head entirely inside the most important part of the deltoid ligament where all the movement is taking place. When the screw can be used less vertically, in large fragments, it does not lie so intimately inside the axis of motion in the ligament.

The only justification for the operative treatment of a Pott's fracture is an absolutely perfect 'hair-line' reposition of the fragments with screws lying quite clear of the articular surfaces; anything less than this constitutes meddlesome surgery and the results are likely to be worse than moderate defects of conservative treatment for which nature has a compensating mechanism. It is not sufficiently realised by those beginning careers as fracture surgeons how extremely difficult the operative treatment of an ankle fracture can be if it entails anything more than the simple fixation of the medial malleous. Even with X-ray control and the ankle open for an hour or two the operator may still be dissatisfied with the result. The difficulty in operating on an ankle fracture is not unlike the difficulty in making an accurate amendment to a carbon copy in a typewriter: it is the simplest thing in the world to open the sheets of paper and to see just where the new impression ought to fall, but when the sheets are again applied to each other the making of the impression has in it an element of chance and more often than not is slightly out of register.

Slipping of the Reduction

It would be very helpful if criteria could be found for the cases which could safely be left under conservative care and for those which should be operated on without undue delay. The following points may help:

1. The slipping of a Pott's fracture usually starts within a week of the reduction, and probably within three or four days. Spontaneous lateral displacement of the talus after reduction is probably caused by soft tissues incarcerated between the medial malleolus and the tibia. In the 'reduced' position these soft tissues (including even the tendon of tibialis posterior) are compressed at the time when the first post-reduction X-ray is made. After three or four days the soft parts may swell or reassert some natural elasticity and so push the talus laterally—even in a non-weight-bearing plaster. It frequently happens that if the immediate post-reduction X-ray is satisfactory, the second check radiograph may not be taken until two or three weeks later, and if a slip has occurred the ankle will have been in an unsatisfactory position for the greater part of this time. *The most important X-ray after the closed reduction of a Pott's fracture is one taken towards the end of the first week, because then it is still not too late to achieve a perfect result if operation on the medial malleolus is undertaken forthwith.*

2. A Pott's fracture which is likely to stay in the reduced position under closed treatment should never need force to secure reduction. Great force indicates that soft parts are being compressed and forced into an unnatural position and will later force the talus out of the mortice. If the reduced position cannot be held under the force of gravity alone with the limb in the position indicated in Fig. 201 there is no point in forcing a closed reduction, and the medial malleolus should be explored forthwith to remove obstructing soft parts.

3. An imperfect reduction of the medial malleolus (but one which would be acceptable were it not to deteriorate) suggests that soft parts may be compressed in the fracture gap, and this appearance should be regarded with suspicion. This is perhaps another way of saying the same thing as (2) in that this imperfection might be masked if great force had been used during reduction. By contrast, a very perfect reduction of the medial malleolus, easily obtained, indicates that no soft tissues are incarcerated and that conservative treatment can be pursued confidently.

4. In cases where initially there has been gross displacement the chance of soft tissue being incarcerated in the gap of the medial malleolus is always much

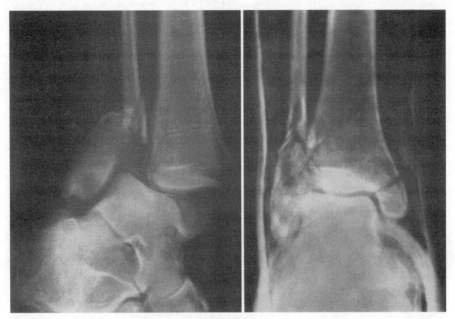

FIG. 215

Gross initial displacement in Pott's fracture increases the possibility of incarceration of soft structures; a perfect reduction such as this, obtained easily by gravity and without undue force, indicates that it can be held conservatively, but with this degree of initial displacement it would be safer to screw the medial malleolus.

greater than with lesser degrees of initial displacement (Fig. 215). Fixation of the medial malleolus is therefore advised if the initial displacement has been gross.

5. Weight-bearing should not be permitted, in fractures which were severely displaced, in less than six to eight weeks, when the plaster should be changed into a new close-fitting plaster before weight-bearing is allowed.

INDEX

THE JOHN CHARNLEY TRUST

AIMS

WHEN Sir John Charnley died in August 1982 and the tributes had been paid to his outstanding pioneering work in the field of total hip replacement, it would have been easy to regard his life and contributions to orthopædic surgery as a matter of history.

Fortunately, his widow, Lady Charnley, was convinced that she had a duty to ensure that a major piece of research that he had commenced should be completed and that his memory be perpetuated through fellowships. Lady Charnley consulted friends and colleagues who had known him, and it was decided to form a charitable trust in his name, to launch an initial appeal to Sir John's former patients and to obtain sponsorship from certain companies with whom he had worked on the many aspects of total hip replacement. Such was the quality of his former patients' experience following the replacement of their defective hip joint by one of his desgns that they, and the sponsoring companies, responded generously.

The aims of the Trust are:

1. The promotion of research into the field of human joint replacement and in particular that of Low Friction Arthroplasty of the hip.
2. The creation of research fellowships and the making of grants to enable young orthopædic surgeons to visit centres of excellence in orthopædic surgery.
3. The sponsorship of lectures, seminars and conferences to further the technique of Low Friction Arthtroplasty pioneered by Sir John Charnley.

The evaluation of the success and failure of any joint replacement can only be obtained by meticulous long term follow up and comparison between different types of prostheses. At present, a cemented Charnley prothesis is considered the Gold Standard and now has a 30-year follow up. Any modifications or improvements must be rigorously compared and early warning of failure must be published to avoid disasters. Research has shown that a follow up period of less than seven years has little value as a prediction of longevity. The Trust requires donations to fund this research as well as continued applications from orthopædic surgeons.

★   ★   ★

Since Sir John died in August 1982, his widow, Lady Charnley, has worked tirelessly to continue the work he started though *The John Charnley Trust*, which has made charitable payments of over £750,000 to date. If you would like to receive further information about the Trust's work, or if you are able to make a donation, please contact:

The Secretaries of The John Charnley Trust,
c/o McMillan & Co., Manor House,
Carr Lane, Croston,
PRESTON, PR5 7RE
U.K.